Tarascon Emergency Department Quick Reference Guide

From the publishers of the *Tarascon Pocket Pharmacopoeia®*

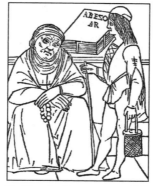

D. Brady Pregerson, MD

Editor-in-Chief, EMresource.org
Attending Physician
Department of Emergency Medicine
Cedars-Sinai Medical Center
Los Angeles, CA

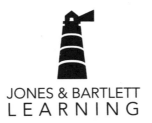

JONES & BARTLETT
LEARNING

World Headquarters
Jones & Bartlett Learning
40 Tall Pine Drive
Sudbury, MA 01776
978-443-5000
info@jblearning.com
www.jblearning.com

Jones & Bartlett Learning Canada
6339 Ormindale Way
Mississauga, Ontario L5V 1J2
Canada

Jones & Bartlett Learning International
Barb House, Barb Mews
London W6 7PA
United Kingdom

Jones & Bartlett Learning books and products are available through most bookstores and online booksellers. To contact Jones & Bartlett Learning directly, call 800–832-0034, fax 978–443-8000, or visit our website, www.jblearning.com.

Substantial discounts on bulk quantities of Jones & Bartlett Learning publications are available to corporations, professional associations, and other qualified organizations. For details and specific discount information, contact the special sales department at Jones & Bartlett Learning via the above contact information or send an email to specialsales@jblearning.com.

The authors, editor, and publisher have made every effort to provide accurate information. However, they are not responsible for errors, omissions, or for any outcomes related to the use of the contents of this book and take no responsibility for the use of the products and procedures described. Treatments and side effects described in this book may not be applicable to all people; likewise, some people may require a dose or experience a side effect that is not described herein. Drugs and medical devices are discussed that may have limited availability controlled by the Food and Drug Administration (FDA) for use only in a research study or clinical trial. Research, clinical practice, and government regulations often change the accepted standard in this field. When consideration is being given to use of any drug in the clinical setting, the healthcare provider or reader is responsible for determining FDA status of the drug, reading the package insert, and reviewing prescribing information for the most up-to-date recommendations on dose, precautions, and contraindications, and determining the appropriate usage for the product. This is especially important in the case of drugs that are new or seldom used.

Library of Congress Cataloging-in-Publication Data
Pregerson, D. Brady.
   Tarascon emergency department quick reference guide / D. Brady Pregerson.
      p. ; cm.
   Emergency department quick reference
   Includes bibliographical references and index.
   ISBN-13: 978-0-7637-8789-9
   ISBN-10: 0-7637-8789-2
1. Emergency medicine—Handbooks, manuals, etc.   2. Hospitals—Emergency services—Handbooks, manuals, etc. I. Title.   II. Title: Emergency department quick reference.
   [DNLM: 1. Emergency Service, Hospital—Handbooks. WX 39]
   RC86.8.P74 2011
   616.02'5—dc22   2010036988

6048

Printed in the United States of America
14 13 12 11 10   10 9 8 7 6 5 4 3 2 1

All efforts have been made to assure the accuracy of this book. However, the accuracy and completeness of information in the *Tarascon Emergency Department Quick Reference Guide* cannot be guaranteed. This book may contain typographical errors and omissions. Its contents are to be used as a guide only; healthcare professionals should use sound clinical judgment and individualize therapy in each patient care situation. Patient interaction and communication is an art that requires clinical intuition, experience, and good judgment. Cultural, linguistic, and individual factors play a part both in the message given and received. This book is meant to serve as a 'field guide' only and is not a substitute for a well-trained medical interpreter. This book is sold without warranties of any kind, express or implied. The publisher, editors, author, and reviewers disclaim any liability, loss, or damage caused by the contents.

Production Credits
Senior Acquisitions Editor: Nancy Anastasi Duffy
Editorial Assistant: Sara Cameron
Associate Production Editor: Laura Almozara
Marketing Manager: Rebecca Rockel
V.P., Manufacturing and Inventory Control: Therese Connell
Composition: Newgen
Cover Design: Scott Moden
Cover Image: Reproduced from Johannes de Ketham. Fasiculo de medecina. Venice: Zuane & Gregorio di Gregorii, 1494.
          Photo Courtesy of National Library of Medicine.
Cover Printing: Cenveo
Printing and Binding: Cenveo

CONTENTS

CONTRIBUTORS	vi
HIPPOCRATIC OATH: A SUMMARY	vi
INTRODUCTION: HOW TO USE THIS BOOK	vii
ERRATA UPDATES AND READER RESPONSIBILITIES	vii
ABBREVIATIONS	viii

1. HISTORY AND THE PHYSICAL EXAM — 1
The History — 1
Physical Exam — 4
2. DIAGNOSTIC TESTS: EKGs, LAB, AND IMAGING — 17
Tests: Utility, Cost, Risks, and Adjustments — 17
EKG — 18
Lab — 30
Radiation Risks from Diagnostic Imaging — 45
X-rays — 47
Ultrasound — 53
CT Scans — 61
Nuclear Medicine Tests — 65
Other Cardiovascular Imaging — 66
3. PROCEDURES — 69
Basics — 69
Airway — 70
Breathing — 74
Circulation — 77
Abdomen — 81
Genitourinary — 82
Obstetrics/Gynecology — 83
Central Nervous System — 84
Eyes — 86
Ears, Nose, and Throat — 87
Compartment Syndrome and Tendonitis — 88
Arthrocentesis and Joint Injections — 89
Dislocations — 90
Fractures and Splints — 92
Lacerations — 93
Incision & Drainage, Excisions — 98
Procedural Sedation Basics — 99

4. DIAGNOSES, DISPOSITION, AND LAWS — 101
Diagnoses and Pitfalls — 101
Disposition — 103
California State and Federal Law — 110
5. RISK MANAGEMENT, MED-LEGAL, AND BILLING — 113
Risk Management — 113
Med-Legal — 117
Billing — 119
6. ACADEMICS, TEAMWORK, AND WELL-BEING — 121
Medical Literature Basics — 121
Teamwork in the ED — 123
Career, Wellness, and Finance — 125
Random Thoughts — 129
7. RESUSCITATION — 131
Adult Resuscitation — 131
Shock and Pressors — 135
Highlights of Critical Care Drugs — 136
Pediatric Resuscitation — 137
Neonatal Resuscitation — 139

APPENDICES — 140
Common Medical Terms Translated — 140
Quick Reference — 174
RESOURCES — 177
Selected Resources — 177
Personal "In a Pinch" Specialist Phone List — 178
INDEX — 179

CONTRIBUTORS

Pravin Acharya, MD
Jonathan Crisp, MS, MD
Joanne Davis, MD
Kevin Dean, MD
Becky C. Doran, MD
Brian R. Floyd, MD
Suzanne Geimer, RN-CN3
Vanessa L. Greene, MD
David Gutkin, DO
Corey R. Heitz, MD
Dana Hendry, MD
Josh Hui, MD
Preeti Jois-Bilowich, MD

Taylor Kallas, MD
Rene Kenney, PA-C
Dan Kopp, MD
Todd Larsen, MD
Lisa Lowe, MD
David T. Matero, MD
Brian McCambley, MS, PA-C
Anthony Medak, MD
Jessica Ngo, MD
Heather Pregerson, PA-C
Nathan Rhodes, MD
Teresa Wu, MD
Nancy Vasquez, RN, LNC

HIPPOCRATIC OATH: A SUMMARY

TRADITIONAL VERSION
Respect your teachers.
Pass on your knowledge.
Protect your patients from harm and injustice.
Do not assist in suicide or abortion.
Do not use the knife.
Do not become intimate with patients.
Protect your patients' confidentiality.

MODERN VERSION
Pledge your life to the service of others.
Place your patients' interests before your own.
Treat all people equally.
Respect the patient's right to make health decisions.
Continue to improve the care you give.
Try to prevent as well as cure disease.
Impart your medical knowledge to others.

1. Be prepared for brevity. This book evolved from super-distilled notes put together to study for oral exams. Sometimes the basics are left out and the focus is on clinically essential but overlooked aspects of care. Use this book as a study guide or to double-check yourself during a shift.
2. Familiarize yourself with the Table of Contents. Topic arrangement tends to be alphabetical.
3. Letters in quotations (i.e., "CUE") signify a mnemonic (and text within parentheses represents something occasional or optional or is a sublist).
4. There are many abbreviations. Learn the symbols in the following table before diving in; it will help.

Important Symbols and Numerical Abbreviations

Arrows	↑ or ^ : rises, elevation, or high		↓: decreases, drop, or low	
	> : more common than or leads to		>> : much greater than	
	→ : causes, leads to			
Letters	ū or u: usually	ĉ or c: with š or s: without		x: times, for, or except
	a: ante (before)	p: post (after) w/: with		
Numbers	CXR: 60/10 (or 60%/10%) For a test: 1st number: sensitivity; 2nd number: specificity			
	CXR: 95 (or 95%) For a test: if only one number: sensitivity			
	N/V: 50 (or 50%) For a symptom/sign: the percent of time it is present			
Other	°: degree (1°: primary)		≡: by definition α: alpha	
	Δ: change, triad, delta		β: beta	
	( ): optional or occasional		': minutes µ: microgram	
	?: uncertainty		2PD: Two-point discrimination	

ERRATA UPDATES AND READER RESPONSIBILITIES

Please be sure to subscribe to the Tarascon Monthly Dose eNewsletter at www.tarascon.com in order to be notified when any new errata to this book are discovered. Please also submit any possible errors that you discover or any other suggestions for improvements by email to editor@tarascon.com.

A

a: Before (ante)
A: Anorexia
Aa: Alveolar–arterial gradient
AA: African American
Ab: Antibody
abdo: Abdominal
ABEM: American Board of Emergency Medicine
ABG: Arterial Blood Gas
ABI: Ankle Brachial Index
abnl: Abnormal
ABX: Antibiotics
AC: Activated Charcoal
ACEP: American College of Emergency Physicians
ACh: Acetyl-Choline
ACI: After Care Instructions
ACS: Acute Coronary Syndrome
AFB: Acid Fast Bacilli (TB)
Afib: Atrial Fibrillation
AFL: Air Fluid Level
Ag: Antigen
AGE: Air Gas Embolism or Acute GastroEnteritis
AGN: Acute GlomeruloNephritis
AH: Auditory Hallucination
AHA: American Heart Association
AHRQ: Agency for Healthcare Research and Quality
AI: Aortic Insufficiency
AIN: Acute Interstitial Glomerulonephritis
AIVR: Acceller IdioVentricular Rhythm
AKA: Also Known As or Alcoholic Keto-Acidosis
alb: Albumin
ALC: Absolute Lymphocyte Count
alk phos: Alkaline phosphatase
ALOC: Altered Level Of Consciousness
ALS: Amyotrophic Lateral Sclerosis
Alt: Alternate Rx
ALZ: Alzheimer's disease
AMI: Acute Myocardial Infarction
amio: Amiodarone
AMS: Altered Mental Status
amy: Amylase

ANC: Absolute Neutrophil Count
ANS: Autonomic Nervous System
ant: Anterior
antichol: Anticholinergic
anx: Anxiety
AP: Abdominal Pain
APAP: Acetaminophen
APB: Abductor Pollicis Brevis
APD: Afferent Pupillary Defect
APLS: AntiPhosphoLipid Syndrome
appy: Appendicitis
AR: Aortic Regurgitation
ARB: Angiotensin Receptor Blocker
ARF: Acute Rheumatic Fever or Acute Renal Failure
AS: Aortic Stenosis
ASA: Aspirin
ASD: Atrial Septal Defect
Asp: Aspirate or Aspiration
aSx: Asymptomatic
AT3: AntiThrombin 3 deficiency
ATN: Acute Tubular Necrosis
ATX: Atelectasis
Av: Average
AV: Arterio-Venous
AVB: AtrioVentricular Block
AVM: ArterioVenous Malformation
AW: AirWay
Ax: Associated (with)

B

B: Bilateral
barbs: Barbiturates
BB: Beta Blocker
BBB: Bundle Branch Block
b/c: Because
BCG: Bacille Calmette-Guérin, TB vaccine
BCx: Blood Culture
benzo: Benzodiazepine
BER: Benign Early Repolarization
BHT: Blunt Head Trauma
bic, bicarb: Bicarbonate

bilat: Bilateral
bili: Bilirubin
BiPAP: Bilevel Positive Airway Pressure
BM: Bowel Movement
BME: BiManual Exam
BMP: Basic Metabolic Panel
BPH: Benign Prostatic Hypertrophy
BVM: Bag Valve Mask
Bx: Biopsy

C

ĉ: With
c: With
Ca: Calcium
CA: Cancer
CAD: Coronary Artery Disease
CAPD: Continuous Ambulatory Peritoneal Dialysis
CBL: Cerebellum
CBZ: Carbamazepine
CCB: Calcium Channel Blocker
Cef: Cephalosporin
CHF: Congestive Heart Failure
chole: Cholecystitis
chrich: Chrichothyroidotomy
CICU: Cardiac ICU
CK: Creatinine Kinase
CM: Cardiac Monitor, CardioMyopathy, CardioMegaly, or CardiacMotion
CMA: Continuously Monitored Area
CML: Chronic Myelogenous Leukemia
CMT: Cervical Motion Tenderness
CMV: CytoMegaloVirus
CN: Cranial Nerve or CyaNide
CNS: Central Nervous System
CO: Carbon monoxide
COD: Cause Of Death
coke: Cocaine
Comp: Compensation or Complications
conc: Concentration
contam: Contamination
Co-Op: Cooperative
CoP: Conditions of Participation
COPD: Chronic Obstructive Pulmonary Disease

cor: Cardiac/heart
COU: Cardiac Observation Unit = Telemetry
coum: Coumadin
CP: Chest Pain or Cerebral Palsy
CPA: Cerebro-Pontine Angle
CPM: Central Pontine Myelinolysis
CPS: Child Protective Services
Cr: Creatinine
CR: Capillary Refill
CRF: Chronic Renal Failure
crine: EndoCrine
c/s: Caesarian Section
CS: Compartment Syndrome
CSF: CerebroSpinal Fluid
CT: Computed Tomography
CTA: CT Angiogram
CTD: Connective Tissue Disease
CV: CardioVascular
CVC: Central Venous Catheter
CVD: Collagen Vascular Disease
CVST: Cavernous Vein Sinus Thrombosis
Cx: Cause or Culture
CZI: Crystaline Zinc Insulin

D

d: Days
DA: Dopamine
D/C or DC: Discharge
DDx: Differential diagnosis
defib: Defibrillation
depo: Deposition
dex: Dexamethasone
DFA: Direct Flourescent Antibody
DHS: Department of Health Services
di: Diarrhea
DI: Diabetes Insipidus
DIC: Disseminated Intravascular Coagulation
dif: Difference or Differential
Dig: Digoxin
DIP: Distal InterPhalangeal
dispo: Disposition
DKA: Diabetic Keto-Acidosis

dlc: Dislocation
DM: Diabetes Mellitus
d/o: Disorder
DP: Dorsalis Pedis
DPL: Diagnostic Peritoneal Lavage
DPT: Diphtheria Pertussis Tetanus
dT: Diphtheria-Tetanus vaccine
DTR: Deep Tendon Reflex
duod: Duodenum
Dur: Duration
DVT: Deep Vein Thrombosis
d/w: Discussed with
dysr: Dysrhythmia
dz: Disease

E

E: Edema
EAST: Elevated Arm Stress Test
EBL: Estimated Blood Loss
EBV: Epstein Barr Virus
ED: Emergency Department
EDTA: EthyleneDiamineTetraacetic Acid
EES: Erythromycin EStolate
EF: Ejection Fraction
EGD: EsophaGoDuodenoscopy
EGDT: Early Goal-Directed Therapy
EHL: Extensor Hallucis Longus
EIA: Enzyme ImmunoAssay
EJ: External Jugular
EKG: Electrocardiogram
EMG: ElecroMyeloGram
EMLA: Eutectic Mixture Local Anesthetic
EMS: Emergency Medical Services
EMT: Emergency Medical Technician
ENT: Ear, Nose, and Throat
e/o: Evidence or
EOMs: ExtraOcular Movements
eos: Eosinophils
EP: Emergency Physician
EPAP: Expiratory Positive Airway Pressure
epi: Epinephrine
EPL: Extensor Policis Longus
ER: Emergency Room

ESLD: End-Stage Liver Disease
esof: Esophagus
esp: Especially
ESR: Erythrocyte Sedimentation Rate
ESRD: End-Stage Renal Disease
EtOH: Ethanol
ETT: EndoTracheal Tube

F

F: Fever
Fab: Fab fragment
FB(O): Foreign Body (Obstruction)
FDIC: Federal Deposit Insurance Corporation
FDS: Flexor Digitorum Superficialis
FDWS: First Dorsal Web Space
FENa: Fractional Excretion sodium
FH: Family History
FHM: Fetal Heart Monitor
FHR: Fetal Heart Rate
fib: Fibrillation
FN: False Negative
FNF: Finger–Nose–Finger test
FOV: Fields Of Vision
FP: False Positive
FSG: Finger Stick Glucose
FVC: Forced Vital Capacity
fx: Fracture
fxn: Function

G

G6PD: Glucose 6-Phosphate Deficiency
GAS: Group A Streptococcal Disease
GBS: Guillain Barre Syndrome or Group B Strep
GC: GonoCoccus/gonorrhea
gen: General
GERD: GastroEsophageal Reflux Dz
GI: GastroIntestinal
GIB: GI Bleed
GIK: Glucose Insulin K+
glu: Glucose
gluc: Gluconate
GN: GlomeruloNephritis
GR: GenitoRectal

GS: Gram Stain
GSW: Gun Shot Wound
GU: GenitoUrinary

H

H: Hydrogen
H1: Antihistamine type 1
H2: Antihistamine type 2
HA: HeadAche
Hb: Hemoglobin
HBIG: HBV Immune Globulin
HBO: HyperBaric Oxygen
HBr: Hydrogen Bromide
HbS: Sulf-Hemoglobin
HBV: Hepatitis B Virus
HCG: Beta-HCG
HCP: HydroCePhalus
HCTZ: HydroChloroThiaZide
HCV: Hepatitis C Virus
HD: Hemidiaphragm or hemodialysis
hem: Hemorrhage
HF&M: Hand, Foot, and Mouth disease
HLOC: Higher Level Of Care
HM: HistaMine
HMO: Health Maintenance Organization
HOB: Head Of Bed
H&P: History & Physical
HPI: History of Present Illness
HPV: Human PapillomaVirus
HR: Heart Rate
HRT: Hormone Replacement Therapy
HSM: HepatoSplenoMegaly
HSP: Henoch-Schönlein Purpura
HTN: HyperTensioN
HTS: Hypertonic Saline
HTX: HemoThoraX
HUS: Hemolytic Uremic Syndrome
Hx: History

I

i: Incidence
IA: Class 1A antidysrhythmic
IABP: IntraAortic Balloon Pump

IBD: Inflammatory Bowel Disease
IBS: Irritable Bowel Syndrome
ibu: Ibuprofen
ICB: IntraCranial Bleed
I&D: Incision & Drainage
ID: Infectious Disease
idio: Idiopathic
IDU: Injection Drug Use
IgA: Immunoglobulin A
IgG: Immunoglobulin G
IgM: Immunoglobulin M
IHSS: Idiopathic Hypertrophic Subaortic Stenosis
IJ: Internal Jugular
Im: Immunosuppression
imp: Important
inf: Inferior
inflam: Inflammation
INH: Isoniazid
INR: International Normalized Ratio
IO: IntraOsseous
IOP: IntraOcular Pressure
IOS: Index Of Suspicion
IPAP: Inspiratory Positive Airway Pressure
IR: Interventional Radiology
IV: Intravenous
IVC: Inferior Vena Cava
IVCD: IntraVentricular Conduction Delay
IVF: IV Fluid
IVIG: IV ImmunoGlobulin

J

J: Joule
JVD: Jugular Venous Distension
jxn: Junction
jxnl: Junctional

K

k: Kilogram
K: Kilo or Potassium
K+: Potassium
kg: Kilogram
KO: Knocked Out
KS: Kaposi's Sarcoma

L

L: Liter or Liver

Lac: Laceration

LAD: Left Anterior Descending or Left Axis Deviation

LAN: LymphAdeNopathy

Lat: Lateral

LBBB: Left Bundle Branch Block

LCx: Left Circumflex artery

LD50: Lethal Dose in 50%

LE: Lambert Eaton or Leukocyte Esterase

LET: Lidocaine-Epi-Tetracaine

LGIB: Lower GI Bleed

Li: Lithium

LI: Large Intestine

Lido: Lidocaine

lig: Ligament

LLDC: Left Lateral DeCubitus

LLQ: Left Lower Quadrant

LLSA: Lifelong Learning Self Assessment

LMA: Laryngeal Mask Airway

LMP: Last Menstrual Period

LOC: Loss Of Consciousness

LR: Lactated Ringers

LVH: Left Ventricular Hypertrophy

lytes: ElectroLytes

Lz: Lesion

M

m: minutes

M: Murmur

Mag: Magnesium

MAI: Mycobacterium Avium Intracellulare

MAOI: MonoAmine Oxidase Inhibitor

MAST: Military Anti-Shock Trousers

MAT: Multifocal Atrial Tachycardia

max: Maximum

MCA: MotorCycle Accident

mg: milligram

MCP: MetacarpoPhalangeal

MCV: Mean Corpuscular Volume

MD: Medical Doctor

MDAC: Multi-Dose Activated Charcoal

MDM: Medical Decision Making

med: Medication

mEq: MilliEquivalents

metHb: MetHemoglobin

Mg: Magnesium

MG: Myasthenia Gravis

MGC: MeninGoCoccus

MI: Myocardial Infarction

min: Minimum

misc: Miscellaneous

ml: Milileters

MM: Multiple Myeloma

MMR: Measles, Mumps, and Rubella

MMSE: Mini-Mental Status Exam

mo: Month

MOF: MultiOrgan Failure

MR: May Repeat

MRSA: Methicillin Resistant Staph Aureus

MS: Multiple Sclerosis, MediaStinum, or Morphine Sulfate

MSE: Medical Screening Exam

msec: Millisecond

mSv: MilliSieverts (radiation dose)

MT: Metatarsal

MTX: MethoTreXate

MVP: Mitral Valve Prolapse

N

NAC: N-Acetyl Cysteine

narcs: Narcotics

NAT: Non-Accidental Trauma

ND: Non-Displaced

NE: NorEpinephrine

neb: Nebulized medication

neg: Negative

NG: NasoGastric

NICU: Neonatal Intensive Care Unit

NIF: Negative Inspiratory Force

nl: Normal

NMJ: NeuroMuscular Junction

NMS: Neuroleptic Malignant Syndrome

NNT: Number Needed to Treat

NNTH: Number Needed to Harm

NO: No (= a pitfall)
NPO: Nil Per Os; Nothing by mouth
NRB: Non Re-Breather
NS: Normal Saline or Night Sweats
NSAID: NonSteroidal Anti-Inflammatory Drug
NSTWC: Non-Specific T-Wave Changes
NTG: NiTroGlycerine
NTP: NiTroPrusside
N/V: Nausea, Vomiting
NV: NeuroVascular
NVI: NeuroVascular Intact
NWB: Non-Weight Bearing

O

OA: OsteoArthritis
OB: Obstetric/pregnant
obs: Observation
occ: Occasionally
OCP: Oral Contraceptive Pill
OGT: Oro Gastric Tube
OI: Opportunistic Infection
OM: Otitis Media
On: Onset
OOC: Out Of Control
O&P: Ova & Parasites
OP: OroPharyngeal
OR: Operating Room/Surgery
ORIF: Open Reduction Internal Fixation
ORT: Oral Rehydration Therapy
osms: Osmolality
OSVS: OrthoStatic Vital Signs
OTC: Over The Counter

P

p: Post (after)
p450: p450 drug interactions
PAC's: Premature Atrial Contractions
PAN: PolyArteritis Nodosa
Pav: Pavulon
PCKD: PolyCystic Kidney Disease
PCR: Polymerase Chain Reaction
PCV: PolyCythemia Vera
PCWP: Pulmonary Capillary Wedge Pressure

PDA: Patent Ductus Arteriosis
PE: Pulmonary Embolism
peds: Pediatrics
PEP: Post-Exposure Prophylaxis
PFO: Patent Foramen Ovale
pheo: Pheochromocytoma
phos: Phosphorous
PHTN: Pulmonary HTN
PIH: Pregnancy-Induced HTN
PIP: Proximal InterPhalangeal or
    Peak Inspiratory Pressure
PLEX: PLasma EXchange
PMC: PneuMoCoccus
PMD: Primary Medical Doctor
PMH: Past Medical History
PMN: PolyMorphic Neutrophil
PNA: PNeumoniA
PNH: Paroxysmal Nocturnal Hematuria
PNS: Peripheral Nervous System
POC: Point Of Care (lab test)
POOP: Pain Out Of Proportion
pos: Positive
post: Posterior
PPD: Purified Protein Derivative, TB test
PPI: Proton Pump Inhibitor
Ppt: Precipitant
PPV: Positive Pressure Ventilation
PRBC: Packed Red Blood Cells
pred: Prednisone
PRICE: Protect, Rest, ICe, Elevate
prn: Pro re nata; as needed
prob: Probability
Pseud: Pseudomonas
PSH: Past Surgical History
PSI: Passenger Space Intrusion or Pounds per Square Inch
PTA: PeriTonsillar Abscess
PTH: ParaThyroid Hormone
PTX: PneumoThoraX
PUD: Peptic Ulcer Disease
PVD: Peripheral Vascular Dz
PVR: Post-Void Residual
p/w: Presents with
Px: Prognosis

Q

q, Q: Each or Q wave
QD: Daily
QID: Four times a day
Quin: Quinolone

R

RA: Rheumatoid Arthritis or Right Atrium
RAD: Reactive Airway Dz, Right Axis Deviation, or Radiation Absorbed Dose
r/b: Relieved by
RBBB: Right Bundle Branch Block
RBC: Red Blood Cell
RCA: Right Coronary Artery
RCT: Random Controlled Trial
RDW: RBC Distribution Width
rec: Recommendation
resps: Respirations
retroP: RetroPeritoneal
RF: Risk Factors
RGR: Rebound, Guarding, Rigidity
RHD: Rheumatic Heart Disease
RI: Renal Insufficiency
RICE: Rest, Ice, Compression, Elevate
RLQ: Right Lower Quadrant
RMSF: Rocky Mountain Spotted Fever
Roc: Rocuronium
roids: Steroids
ROPA: Regional Organ Procurement Agency
ROS: Review Of Systems
ROSC: Return of Spontaneous Circulation
RPA: RetroPharyngeal Abscess
RR: Respiratory Rate
RSD: Reflex Sympathetic Dystrophy
RSI: Rapid Sequence Induction
RSV: Respiratory Syncytial Virus
RT: Respiratory Therapist
RTA: Renal Tubular Acidosis
RTED: Return to Emergency Department
RTER: Return to Emergency Room
RUG: Retrograde UrethroGram
RUQ: Right Upper Quadrant
RV: Right Ventricle
RVMI: Right Ventricular MI

RVU: Relative Value Unit
Rx: Treatment
rxn: Reaction

S

$\bar{s}$: Without
s: Without or seconds
SAAG: Serum Ascites Albumin Gradient
SAC: Short Arm Cast
SAEM: Society for Academic Emergency Medicine
sarc: Sarcoid
SARS: Severe Acute Respiratory Syndrome
SAT: Syringe Aspiration Technique
SBE: Subacute Bacterial Endocarditis
SBP: Systolic Blood Pressure
SCC: Squamous Cell Carcinoma
SCM: SternoCleidoMastoid
SDE: SubDural Empyema
SDH: SubDural Hematoma
Seb-K: Seborrheic Keratosis
seds: Sedative
sg: Specific gravity
SH: Social History
SI: Sacrolliac, Suicidal Ideate, or Small Intestine
Sides: Side Effects
SIPC: Securities Investor Protection Corporation
SJS: Steven Johnson Syndrome
SLC: Short Leg Cast
SLE: Systemic Lupus Erythematosis
SLR: Straight Leg Raise
SLUDGE: Salivation Lacrimation Urination Defecation GI upset Emesis
SLWC: Short Leg Walking Cast
SMA: Superior Mesenteric Artery
Sn: (physical exam) Sign
SNF: Skilled Nursing Facillity
SOB: Short Of Breath
SR: Sustained Release
sroid: Steroid
SSRI: Serotonin Selective Reuptake Inhibitor
SSS: Sick Sinus Syndrome
ST: Sore Throat
ST↑: Sore Throat elevation

STS: Soft Tissue Swelling
succ: SuccinylCholine
sup: Superior or supinate
sux: Succinylcholine
SW: Social Worker
Sx: Symptom
sym: Symmetric
synd: Syndrome
Sz: Seizure

T

T: Temperature
t ½ : Half Life
TA: Temporal Arteritis
TAC: Tetracaine Adrenaline Cocaine
tach: Tachycardia
TACO: Transfusion Associated Circulatory Overload
Tamp: Tamponade
TB: Tuberculosis
Tberg: Trendelenberg
T & C: Type & Cross
TCA: TriCyclic Antidepressant
TCN: TetraCycliNe
TEE: TransEsophageal Echo
Tele: Telemetry
temp: Temperature
TEN: ToxEpidermal Necrolysis
thy: Thyroid
TIBC: Total Iron Binding Capacity
tic: DiverTICulitis
TM: Tympanic Membrane
tob: Tobacco
tox: Toxicology
toxo: Toxoplasmosis
TPN: Total Parenteral Nutrition
TPTX: Tension PneumoThoraX
TRA: Traumatic Ruptured Aorta
TRALI: Transfusion Related Acute Lung Injury
trich: Trichomonas
trop: Troponin
TSH: Thyroid Stimulating Hormone
TSS: Toxic Shock Syndrome
TT: Tetanus Toxoid

TTP: Tender To Palpation
Tyl: Tylenol

U

ū: Usually
u: Usually or units
UA: Unstable Angina
UC: Ulcerative Colitis or
    Uterine Contraction
UGI: Upper GI
ULN: Upper Limit of Normal
UNa: Urine Sodium
unk: Unknown
UOP: Urine OutPut
URI: Upper Respiratory Infection
US: UltraSound
UTZ: Ultrasound (used at USC)
UU: Ureaplasma Urealyticum

V

V: Vomiting
Vag: Vaginal
vanco: Vancomycin
VB: Vaginal Bleed
VDRL: Venereal Disease Research Lab
VH: Visual Hallucinations
Vit: Vitamin
vol: Volume
VRE: Vanco Resistant Enterococcus
vs.: Versus
VSD: Ventricular Septal Defect
VSUS: Vitals Signs UnStable
VT: Ventricular Tachycardia
vWD: von Willebrand's Disease
VZV: Varicella Zoster Virus

W

WBAT: Weight Bear As Tolerated
WBC: White Blood Cell
WBI: Whole Bowel Irrigation
WC: Wound Check
w/d: Withdrawal
wk: Week
WPW: Wolff-Parkinson-White

X

x: Times, for, except, or trans-
XAP: Xylocaine Adrenaline Pontocaine
XR: X-Ray
XRT: X-Ray Therapy

Z

zap: Defibrillate or Cardiovert

Symbols

$\uparrow$: Rises, elevation, or high
$\downarrow$: Decreased
$\rightarrow$: Leads to, causes
$>$: Greater than or leads to
$<$: Less than
$>>$: Much greater than
$<<$: Much less than

α: Alpha
β: Beta
Δ: Delta, change
μ: Microgram

( ): Maybe, consider, or variably
$: Expensive
°: Degree
^: Rises, increased, or high
': Minutes, feet, or decreases
": Seconds or inches
~: Approximately

2PD: 2-Point Discrimination
1°: Primary
2°: Secondary
3°: Tertiary
4°: Quaternary

SECTION 1 ■ HISTORY AND THE PHYSICAL EXAM

THE HISTORY

INTRODUCTIONS AND THE BASICS

■ **Entry/Intro:** Make sure you have the correct patient/chart. Don't let foul personalities affect your decisions. Wash hands in front of patient. Introduce yourself to all in room. Shake hands. History is the most important diagnostic tool as well as key to building a good rapport. Get PMD name. Make good eye contact. Watch people's faces and breathing.

■ **Method:** Talk to the spouse/friend/family member and document it. Note facial expression. Sit down.

■ **Questions:** Open ended: "Tell me about your breathing," rather than "Are you short of breath?" "Tell me more about _____." "What are you most worried about?"

■ **Nurse/EMS:** Always review nursing notes and EMS-run sheet.

HISTORY OF PRESENT ILLNESS

What you do not ask, you will not find out.

■ **"OLD CARTS"**

Onset: Day and time, activity at onset, last time normal

Location: Location of pain, discomfort, or other symptoms

Duration: Duration of each episode, frequency of episodes; have they had this before?

Character: Qualitative description of character of discomfort or symptom

Aggravators and Alleviators: Symptoms affected by activity, position, food, motion,...or random?

Radiation: Have the symptoms radiated to additional areas or migrated to a new area?

Treatment: Have any medications or other treatments been tried?

Significance: Have symptoms impacted lifestyle? Have they been to ED before for same? "When's the last time you had something similar? Rx then? Did you get better?"

■ **Prior Visit:** High risk: Do a more thorough workup. Strongly consider admission, especially if 3rd visit.

■ **Positional:** Worse supine: GERD, pericarditis, CHF, COPD. Other positional: PE can be, pancreatitis better in fetal position

■ **Precipitants:** "SHAFTED" (**S**urgery, **H**ypoxia, **A**nemia/acidosis, **F**ever/ID, **T**rauma, **E**mbryo, **D**ehydration)

PEDIATRIC HISTORY

■ **Epidemics**
  ● *Fall:* Croup, rotavirus. *Winter:* RSV, influenza, VZV, rotavirus. *Spring:* parvovirus, rubella, pertusis. *Summer:* Enterovirus, viral meningitis

■ **History:** "PEDS" (**P**ain [crying?], **P**oop/**P**ee [last, hydration?], **E**nergy, **D**iet [nursing OK?], **S**leep)

■ **Exam:** Hi 5, tone, fontanelle, mouth, hip, skin/rash, cap refill, Moro, suck, feed, interaction

■ **Milestones:** 10d: Cord stump should fall off (if > 21d there is a neutrophil problem); 1 mon: Lift head, track, smile; 4 mon: Grasp, reach, coo, roll; 6 mon: Solids, teeth, then 1/mon

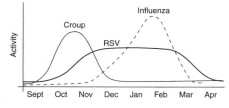

FIGURE 1.1. Seasonal prevalence of common viral infections.

PAST MEDICAL HISTORY

■ **Allergies:** Common are: ASA/NSAID, sulfa, cillin, vanco; dilantin/barbs/CBZ; codeine/MS

■ **Meds:** Meds requiring blood tests? Compliance? New meds? OCP/OTC/herbals? Viagra?
  ● *Dangerous*: Heart (BB/CCB/Dig). Bleed (NSAID/steroid/Coumadin). Sugar (insulin/DM)
  ● *ABX*: Any antibiotics in past month increases risk for resistant organisms, C. dif colitis and fungal ID
  ● *NSAIDs*: Proven for gout and rheumatoid conditions, renal/biliary colic, menstrual cramps. Risks: GI bleed, renal, MI, slowed healing in bones (sprains), mild blood thinning. Alternates: Tylenol, opiates.

■ **Past Surgical History:** Prior surgeries; any recent?

■ **Past Medical History:** Admits, recent surgery, past w/u: TB/RAD, MI, PUD/liver/chole, Sz
  ● *ABX resist*: Hospitalized in past 90d, ABX past 30d, ESRD, in-dwelling line, nursing home, home health

■ **Last:** LMP, dT/Immunizations, Tylenol/ABX, BM/vomit, pain, MD visit, admission

■ **Review of Systems:** GEN-F/C/night sweats/weight loss; CNS-HA/weakness/trauma/vision/hearing/vertigo; CV-chest pain/SOB/cough/syncope; GI-pain/N/V/BMs/melena; GU-dysuria/frequency/polyuria

■ **Screening:** Most effective per SAEM: EtOH, HIV, HTN, adult pneumovax, pediatrician, smoking

■ **Family History:** Sudden death, CAD, CA, etc.

■ **Social History:** "RSTUVW" (**R**ide home?, on the **S**treet, **T**ravel/exposure, **U**se [drugs], **V**iolence, **W**ork)
  ● *Resistance*: Risk for MRSA and Pseudomonas: Healthcare worker or admit in past 3 mon; any ABX or any home health care or SNF in past 3 mon, ESRD
  ● *Travel*: SARS/Avian flu: Asia, Russia, Turkey, Croatia, Kazakhstan
  ● *Heritage*: Avoid sulfa drugs in Southeast Asians as G6PD deficiency very common
  ● *Immigrant*: Eosinophilia usually = worm infection even if O&P repeatedly neg and if in United States for decades. If eosinophilia, do not start steroids without first giving course of albendazole. Asia: Common: Hepatitis B, worms, TB; avoid sulfa drugs because G6PD deficiency very common. Africa: Common: Schistosomiasis, TB.

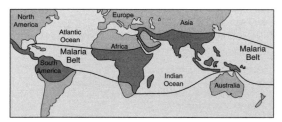

FIGURE 1.2. Rough guide to areas where malaria occurs.

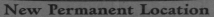

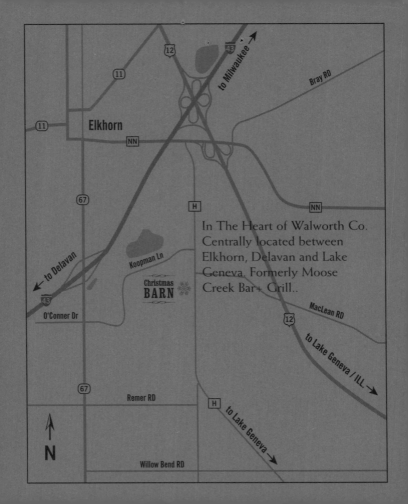

In The Heart of Walworth Co. Centrally located between Elkhorn, Delavan and Lake Geneva. Formerly Moose Creek Bar+ Grill..

HISTORY TAKING IN A FOREIGN LANGUAGE

■ Basics

- *Scope*: 11% U.S. population is foreign born (52% Hispanic, 26% Asian, European 16%, other 6%)
- *Legal*: Official translator is best. Using family can put you at risk medico-legally. If family wants to translate, offer use of interpreter and document family's refusal and reason.

■ Foreign Language Emergencies

How to say "Hello or Good day?"

Arabic:	Salam Alekum
Armenian:	Barev
Farsi:	Sa'lam
French:	Bonjour
German:	Hallo
Hebrew:	Shalom
Japanese:	Konnichi wa
Korean:	Annyong haseyo
Mandarin:	Nĩ hão
Philippino:	Halo
Portuguese:	Bom dia/Boa noit
Russian:	Dobre dein
Spanish:	Hola
Thai:	Sawatdi
Vietnamese:	Kinh Chao

How to say "Where does it hurt?"

Arabic:	Ayna alam
Armenian:	Vortea tsav
Cambodian:	Chu glaina
Cantonese:	Binto toen
Farsi:	Coja dard m'koneh
French:	Ou est douleur
German:	Wo tut es weh
Hebrew:	Eyfo co'ev
Hindi:	Kaha durda
Japanese:	Doko ga itai
Korean:	Odi apayo
Mandarin:	Nani toen
Philippino:	Sa'an masakit
Portuguese:	Onde dor
Russian:	G'de bolna
Spanish:	Donde le duele
Tagalog:	Sa'an masakit
Thai:	Jeb tinae

■ Resources for Foreign Language Translation

- American Sign Language: 800–633-8888
- PALS (Asian and Spanish): 213–553-1818
- Language Line Services: 800–874-9426
- Online Translators: 800–241-1721
- Medical-Leadership: Council http://medicalleadership.org/educational_continued.shtm
- See Appendix: Common Medical Terms Translated (pages 140-173)

PHYSICAL EXAM

VITAL SIGN DECODING

■ **Blood Pressure and DDx's**

- *Technique*: Use correct size cuff, support the arm extended at the level of the heart
- *High BP*: DDx: Spurious, essential HTN, secondary HTN (endocrine, renal artery stenosis, drugs)
- *Low BP*: DDx: (See Shock) pay attention to diastolic BP: JVD? Clear lungs? Murmur? Kussmaul?
- *Wide*: Pulse Pressure: "PAST" (**P**DA, **A**I, **A**V fistula, **S**epsis, **T**SH), coarctation
- *Bilateral BP*: Important to check in hypotension as well: The higher of the two arms is the true BP; 20% of normal people will have a 20 mmHg difference in the SBP
- *Orthostatics*: Don't do if patient already symptomatic: risk > benefit. Stand for 3 min before taking BP. Low sensitivity and specificity. "Positive" if SBP < 90 or drop > 25 or HR ↑ by > 30 (some say 20). DDx: Hypovolemia, autonomic dysfunction, meds, normal variant

■ **Tachycardia and Bradycardia DDx's**

- *Tachycardia*: Traditionally > 100, but > 90 used in sepsis definition and likely abnormal for most people
  ↑: Tox (e.g.: cocaine, antichol), twist (pain or anxiety), TSH/pheo, temp (↑ 1°F > HR ↑ by 10)
  ↓: Blood (anemia, BP, volume, heart), O_2 (PE, CHF), EtOH (withdrawal), glucose↓
- *Bradycardia*: Traditionally < 60, but 50–60 likely normal for most people
  ↑: ↑K, ↑Mg, ↑TSH, ↑Trop, ↑Tox (BB, CCB, clonidine, digoxin, physostigmine, cyanide)
  ↓: ↓Temperature, ↓O_2, ↓glucose, ↓conduction (AVB, SSS)

■ **Respiratory Rate DDx's**

- *Fast RR*: Sepsis, hypoxia, PE, CHF, RAD, ASA, TSH, anxiety, acidosis
- *Slow RR*: Drug (opiate, benzo, etc.), CNS

■ **Pulse Ox**

- *Errors*: Motion, MetHb, COHb, nail polish (esp. blue/green/black), pressors, shock, ↑HR, anemia
- *Lag time*: 10–20 sec for ear, 20–40 sec for finger, 40–80 sec for toe, 5–10 min for COPD

TABLE 1.1.   Hypoxemia

Hypoxemia	Response to 100% O_2	pCO_2	Aa Gradient	DDx
Hypoventilation	Yes	↑	→	Sedation, lung, obstruction, weak
Diffusion defect	Yes	↓	↑	Hepatorenal, other
Shunt	No	↑→	↑	Heart: ASD, TGA, tetralogy Lung: AVM, PNA, hepatopulmonary
VQ mismatch	Yes	↑↓→	↑	Asthma/COPD, atelectasis, CHF, PE
Hypoxia	Yes			CO, altitude, ↓FiO₂

FAHRENHEIT

$°F = (9/5)(°C) + 32$

CENTIGRADE

$°C = (°F–32)/(5/9)$

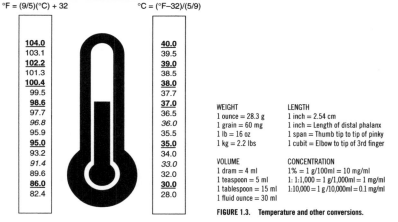

104.0	**40.0**
103.1	39.5
102.2	**39.0**
101.3	38.5
100.4	**38.0**
99.5	37.7
98.6	**37.0**
97.7	36.5
96.8	*36.0*
95.9	35.5
95.0	**35.0**
93.2	34.0
91.4	*33.0*
89.6	32.0
86.0	**30.0**
82.4	28.0

WEIGHT
1 ounce = 28.3 g
1 grain = 60 mg
1 lb = 16 oz
1 kg = 2.2 lbs

LENGTH
1 inch = 2.54 cm
1 inch = Length of distal phalanx
1 span = Thumb tip to tip of pinky
1 cubit = Elbow to tip of 3rd finger

VOLUME
1 dram = 4 ml
1 teaspoon = 5 ml
1 tablespoon = 15 ml
1 fluid ounce = 30 ml

CONCENTRATION
1% = 1 g/100ml = 10 mg/ml
1: 1:1,000 = 1 g/1,000ml = 1 mg/ml
1:10,000 = 1 g /10,000ml = 0.1 mg/ml

FIGURE 1.3.   Temperature and other conversions.

- ■ **Fever and Hypothermia DDx's**
  - ● *Fever*: ID, TSH, CVD, CA (blood, liver, kidney, lung, prost), Tox (NMS, cocaine, antichol), heat stroke.
    Definition: Oral: 37.5°C = 99.5°F, rectal: 38.0°C = 100.4°F (study of healthy volunteers); oral is 0.5°–1°F
    lower than rectal. Armpit is 1°–1.5°F lower than rectal.
  - ● *Hypothermia*: Exposure, sepsis, endocrine, hypoglycemia, Wernicke's, hypothalamus, cord, Meds/tox.

PEDIATRIC EXAM

- ■ **General:** Hi 5, tone, mouth, hip, skin, cap refill, suck, feed, interaction, suck, feed
- ■ **"TICLES"** (Tone, Interactive, Cry strength, Consolable, Cap refill, (L), Eye contact, Suck, Smile)
- ■ **Fontanelle:** Bulging: hydrocephalus, ID, trauma, benign extra-axial fluid of infancy (resolves by 2 yr); Sunken: dehydration
- ■ **Reflexes:** Moro, palmo-mental, glabellar

TABLE 1.2.   Pediatric Vital Signs

Formulae (Age in Years)	0 years	1 year	2 years	4 years	8 years
Weight in kg = 10 + 2 (age) or 4 + (mon/2)	4–10 kg	10 kg	14 kg	18 kg	26 kg
Max normal HR = 170 – 10 (age)	170	160	150	130	90
Min normal BP = 70 + 2 (age)	70	72	74	78	86
Max normal RR = 50 – 10 (age): works until 3 yr	30–60	24–40	24–40	22–34	18–30

Formulae worse as age ↑. Every book has different values.
Source: Pregerson DB. *Quick Essentials Emergency Medicine 4.0.* ERPocketbooks.com; 2010:160.

GENERAL ADVICE

- **Hand Washing:** Wash or sanitize before and after patient contact. Alcohol rubs best for most things. Soap and water best for C. dif, influenza A, and probably some others. Use alcohol-based hand rubs and get your pen and stethoscope too (surface wipes too). Wipe down other fomites such as keyboards and phones with surface wipes.

- **Laying on Hands:** The laying on of hands can be therapeutic and builds rapport.

TABLE 1.3.   Physical Exam Summary Chart

System	Basics	Tests and Pertinent Negatives
General	Comfort level	Cooperative, No Acute Distress
	Fluency of speech	Position of Preference
Vitals	Decode vitals	Diastolic Bp, Bilateral Bp
	Trends	Orthostatics
Skin	Diaphoresis, Rash	Track marks, Petecheiae
	Erythema	Turgor
Head/Face	Trauma	Temporal artery tenderness
	Symmetry	Temporal wasting
Eyes	Eoms, Pupils, Iop, Papilledema	Nystagmus, Horner's, Afferentpupillary defect
	Conjunctiva, Venous pulsations	Slit lamp, Fluoresceine, Seidel's test, Visual fields
Ears	TMs, Canals	Facial nerve
	Tragal tenderness	Hemotympanum, Battle sign
Nose	Trauma, Mucous	Symmetry
	Mass	Septal hematoma
Throat	Mass, Exudate, Thrush	Trismus, Stridor, Drooling, Bulging posteriorly
	Erythema	Tenderness
Neck	Supple, Mass	Thyroid scar
	JVD	Lhermitte's sign
Back	CVAT, Straight leg raise test	Focal tenderness
	Scoliosis	Guarding
Lungs	Auscultation, Rales, Wheezing	Egophony, Splinting for PE
	Dullness	Forced expiratory time
Heart	S1, S2, RRR	Murmur of AS affects Rx for chest pain
	Murmur, Rub, Gallop	Hamman's crunch, AI: ? for dissection
Abdomen	AAA, Tenderness	Bruit, Femoral pulses, No pain out of proportion
	Mass, Pulsations, Bowel sounds	Rovsing's, Obturator sign, Psoas sign
	Rebound	Murphy's sign, NG aspirate > 300 ml
GU/GR	Guaiac, Mass	Volition, Anal wink
	Cremasteric reflex	Post-void residual > 50 ml
	Melena: blood, Lead, Bismuth	Bulbocavernosus reflex, Testicle lie
Extremities	Pulses, Edema	Cap refill, Pulse delay
	Rubor	Homan's sign
CNS	Orientation, Cranial nerves	Asterixis, Hallpike, Clonus, Heel-to-shin
	Motor/tone, Sensory, DTR's	Pronator drift, Romberg
	Finger nose, Rapid movement	Sensory extinction, Graphesthesia, Stereognosis
	Nuchal rigidity, Babinski	Jolt accentuation of headache

TABLE 1.4.   Selected Eponymous Exam Signs

Eponym	Exam Finding	Disease
Adson's	Decreased radial pulse with neck turn and breath-hold	Thoracic outlet syndrome
Brudzinski's	Forced neck flexion produces hip + knee flexion	Meningitis
Cheyne-Stokes	Breathing alternates between fast and slow	CNS disease
Chvostek's	Facial spasm elicited by tapping facial nerve	Hypocalcemia
Dance's	Emptiness to palpation in RLQ	Intussusception
de Musset's	Head bobbing with each systole	Aortic insufficiency
Ewart's	Dull to percussion at L scapula	Pericardial effusion
Fathergill's	Abdomen more tender with abdomen tight/sit-up	Muscle strain
Grey Turner's	Flank ecchymosis	Retroperitoneal bleed
Hamman's	Crunching sound with each heartbeat	Pneumomediastinum
Hoffman's	Flicking tip of 3rd finger causes thumb flexion	Upper motor neuron disease
Homan's	Forced dorsiflexion of foot causes calf pain	DVT
Horner's	Ptosis, miosis, anhydrosis (see Figure 1.4)	Sympathetic lesion
Ishihara's	Color blindness cards	Color blindness
Janeway's	Painless red embolic hand lesions	Endocarditis
Kussmaul's	JVD increases with inspiration	Pericardial tamponade
Levine's	Clenched fist over chest (see Figure 1.5)	MI
Murphy's	Inspiratory splint with RUQ pressure	Cholecystitis
Nikolsky's	Lateral pressure on blister causes extension	Pemphigus, TEN, SSSS
Osler's nodes	Tender nodules on palms	Endocarditis
Phalen's	Prolonged wrist flexion causes median nerve paresthesia (see Figure 1.6)	Carpal tunnel syndrome
Pregerson's	Subpatella bulge with knee flexed	Knee effusion
Prehn's	Testicle pain relieved by support	Epididymitis
Psoas	Hip flexion vs. resistance increases abdominal pain	Appendicitis
Quincke's	Nail bed pulsations with pressure	Aortic insufficiency
Romberg's	Falls with eyes closed	Decreased proprioception
Rovsing's	LLQ percussion causes RLQ pain	Appendicitis
Rumpel Leede	Petechiae from capillary leak after tourniquet or BP cuff	Dengue, RMSF, scarlatina
Steinberg	Thumb IP joint can project past ulnar edge of pinky	Marfan's
Thompson's	Calf squeeze does not cause plantar flexion	Achilles tendon rupture
Tinel's	Percussion of median nerve at wrist provokes parasthesia	Carpal tunnel syndrome
Traube's	Pistol shot sound at femoral artery	Aortic insufficiency
Trousseau's	Carpal spasm from BP cuff (may need > systolic x 3 min)	Hypocalcemia
Uhthoff's	Increased body temp causes worsening neuro sx/sn	Multiple sclerosis
Verneuil's	Distal press/percuss causes proximal pain	Fracture
Vircow's	Palpable left supraclavicular lymph node	Pancreatic or GI cancer
Von Graefe's	Lid lag with visual tracking from high to low	Grave's disease
Walker	1st and 5th digit encircling other wrist overlap proximal to DIP	Marfan's
Weber	Tuning fork to mid forehead heard asymmetrically	Hearing deficit
Yerganson's	Pain and weakness with resisted supination	Biceps tendonitis

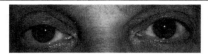

FIGURE 1.4.   Horner's syndrome.

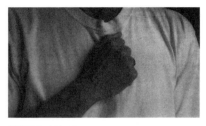

FIGURE 1.5.   Levine sign.

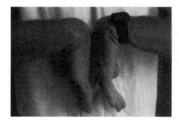

FIGURE 1.6.   Phalen's test.

TABLE 1.5.   Triads of Diseases

Name	Triads
Alport's	Sensorineural deafness, progressive renal failure, and ocular anomalies
Beck's	Hypotension, JVD, and muffled heart tones in pericardial tamponade (a very insensitive triad)
Behcet's	Recurrent oral ulcers, genital ulcers, and iridocyclitis
Charcot's	Fever, jaundice, and RUQ pain in cholangitis (add AMS + shock = Reynold's pentad)
Cushing's	Bradycardia, hypertension, and irregular respirations in increased intracranial pressure
Gradenigo's	6th cranial nerve palsy, ear discharge, and retro-orbital pain in mastoiditis
Horner's	Ptosis, miosis, and anhydrosis in carotid or apical pleural disease
Hutchinson's	Interstitial keratitis, labyrinthine disease, and Hutchinson's teeth in congenital syphilis
Kartagener's	Bronchiectasis, recurrent sinusitis, and situs inversus
O'Donoghue's	Medial collateral and anterior cruciate knee ligament tears plus medial meniscus injury
Pregerson's	Lost prescription, sunglasses, and Toradol allergy in narcotic seeking
Reiter's	Arthritis, urethritis, and conjunctivitis in reactive arthritis (Reiter's disease)
Saint's	Hiatus hernia, colonic diverticula, and cholelithiasis
Sampter's	Asthma, nasal polyposis, and aspirin sensitivity
Virchow's	Trauma, hypercoagulable state, and/or immobility causing venous thromboemblolic disease
Wernicke's	AMS, ataxia, and ophthalmoplegia in thiamin deficiency encephalopathy
Whipple's	Symptoms of hypoglycemia, glucose < 40, and prompt relief on glucose administration

Note: Many triads, though "classical," are not necessarily common.
Source: Pregerson DB. *Quick Essentials Emergency Medicine 4.0.* ERPocketbooks.com; 2010:72.

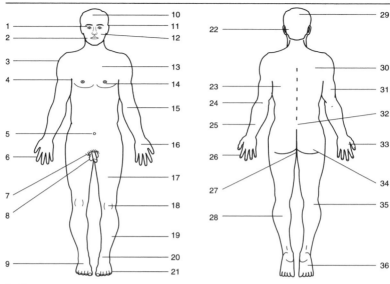

FIGURE 1.7. Derm body map: Certain diseases and common body locations.

1- Eyelids: Xanthalasma, Sty/chalazion, Dermatomyositis
2- Lips and Mouth: Thrush, CA, STD, Lichen planus
3- Shoulder: Melanoma, Acne, Skin CA
4- Axilla: Hidradenitis, Skin tags, Acanthosis
5- Umbilicus: Patent urachus, Hernia, Fungal ID
6- Fingers: Warts, Felon, Osler's, Janeway (See #26)
7- Groin: Fungal infections, STD
8- Genital: STD, Psoriasis, Fungal infections
9- Acral: Neuropathic ulcer, Ischemia, Gout, Ganglion, Tinea
10- Forehead: Acne, Sebaceous hyperplasia, CA, Actinic K
11- Ear: Squamous cell CA, Ramsey-Hunt
12- Cheek: Rosacea, Melasma, SLE, Seborrhea, Eczema
13- Torso: Cherry hemangioma, Telangectasia, Pityriasis
14- Breast: Cyst, CA, Abscess, Fungal
15- Flexural: Eczema, Fungal
16- Palm: Eczema, Syphilis, RMSF, E. multiform, Drug
17- Thigh: Dermatofibroma
18- Extensor: Psoriasis, Poison oak/ivy
19- Shin: Trauma, Ichthiosis, Necrobiosis, E. nodosum
20- Ankle: Stasis Ulcer, Insect bites
21- Toes: Fungal infections, Ingrown nail

22- Behind Ear: Seborrhea, Psoriasis
23- Back—Mid: Café-au-lait, Tinea, Pityriasis (See #30)
24- Extensor: Psoriasis, Gout, Trauma, Bursitis
25- Forearm: Senile purpura, Trauma, CA, Poison oak/ivy
26- Fingers: Paronychia, Pyogenic granuloma, Splinter
27- Perianal: Hemorrhoid, Fissures, Abscess, Fistula, STD
28- Calf: Melanoma, Plantaris tendon rupture, DVT
29- Scalp: Allopecia, Ringworm, Pilar cyst, Discoid lupus
30- Back—Top: Melanoma, CA, Lipoma, Seb-K (See #23)
31- Tricep: Keratosis pilaris, Poison oak/ivy
32- Back—Low: Pilonidal, Mongolian spot (See #23, 30)
33- Hand: Dorsum: Solar keratosis, CA, Ganglion
34- Buttock: Abscess, Acne, Fistula, STD, HSV (See #27)
35- Flexural: Eczema, Baker's cyst
36- Sole: Veruca, Tinea pedis, Drug, Pemphigoid, SBE

OTHER
Dependent: Petechiae, HSP, Venous insufficiency
In Prior Scar: Sarcoid
Mucosal: Lichen planus, HF&M, HSV, Syphilis, Apthous
    Steven-Johnson Syndrome

EYE EXAM

■ Pupils

Check pupils in bright and dim light. Physiologic anisocoria < 3 mm: 20%

- *Horner's causes*: Lung: Pancoast. Neck: Dissection/trauma/OA/ID, nodes. Head: CVA, CBL bleed, cluster HA.
- *Mydriasis*: Unilateral: Trauma, Adie = tonically dilated, CN₃ Either: Chemical: plants or eye drops: Naphcon, etc. (no change w/ pilocarpine 0.1%). Bilateral: "BAD CAT" (**B**otulism, **A**ntichol, **D**iphtheria, **C**ocaine, **A**mphetamine, **T**CA).
- *Miosis*: "PICO" (**P**ons, **P**henothiazine, **I**nsecticide, **C**lonidine, **O**piate). Also: Benzos, barbs, Valproate.

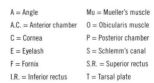

Conditions	Normal Eyes	Adie's Pupil	Argyl-Robertson	Horner's Syndrome	Mydriatic Medicine	Third Nerve Palsy
Normal light	◉ ◉	◉ ◉	◉ ◉	◉ ◉	◉ ◉	◉ ◉
Dim light	◉ ◉	◉ ◉	◉ ◉	◉ ◉	◉ ◉	◉ ◉
Bright light	◉ ◉	◉ ◉	◉ ◉	◉ ◉	◉ ◉	◉ ◉
Accommodation	◉ ◉	◉ ◉	◉ ◉	◉ ◉	◉ ◉	◉ ◉
Pilocarpine	◉ ◉	◉ ◉	◉ ◉	◉ ◉	◉ ◉	◉ ◉

FIGURE 1.8.   Pupillary findings in normal and diseased patients.

■ Nystagmus

- *Peripheral*: Form: Jerk, unidirectional, horizontal or torsional, may have latency. Inhibitors: Gaze fixation or convergence, will fatigue. Enhancers: Gaze in direction of fast phase. Examples include BPPV, labrynthitis.
- *Central*: Form: Jerk or pendular; in direction of gaze; horizontal, vertical, or torsional, no latency. Inhibitors: None. Enhancers: Gaze fixation, does not fatigue. Examples include ethanol, drugs, CVA, MS.

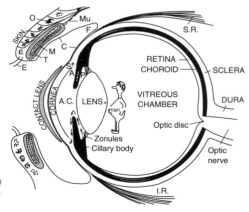

A = Angle
A.C. = Anterior chamber
C = Cornea
E = Eyelash
F = Fornix
I.R. = Inferior rectus
M = Meibomian glands

Mu = Mueller's muscle
O = Obicularis muscle
P = Posterior chamber
S = Schlemm's canal
S.R. = Superior rectus
T = Tarsal plate

FIGURE 1.9.   Eye anatomy.
Adapted from Goldberg S, Ouellette H. *Clinical Anatomy Made Ridiculously Simple*. 3rd ed. Miami, FL: MedMaster; 2007.

CHEST EXAM: THE HEART AND LUNGS

TABLE 1.6.   Abnormal Heart Sounds

Heart Sound	Mnemonic	Causes
S2 (paradoxical)	N/A	↑L-sided volume: LBBB, AS, IHSS
S2 (wide)	N/A	↑R-sided volume: PE, RBBB, ASD, VSD, pulmonic stenosis
S3	Kentucky	CHF, ↑volume, stiff walls, CAD, CM, (cal be normal age < 30)
S4	Tennessee	MI, HTN

Source: Pregerson DB. *Quick Essentials Emergency Medicine 4.0.* ERPocketbooks.com; 2010:67.

TABLE 1.7.   Murmurs

Condition	Murmur Timing	Sounds	Louder With	Other
Aortic stenosis	Systolic	Harsh		Radiates to neck, nl S2
Mitral regurge	Systolic decrescendo	Blowing		Radiates to axilla
Aortic regurge	Diastolic decrescendo	Soft		Wide pulse pressure
Mitral stenosis	Diastolic rumble	Rumble	Precise location	
IHSS	Systolic	Harsh	Valsalva, standing	
Coarctation	Continuous*		Intrascapular	BP arms–legs > 20

*Continuous murmur: Patent ductus, air gas embolism, venous hum, coarctation

Source: Pregerson DB. *Quick Essentials Emergency Medicine 4.0.* ERPocketbooks.com; 2010:67.

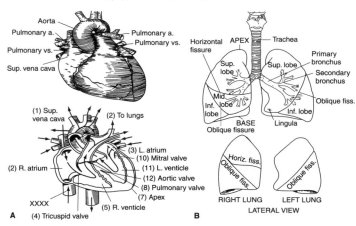

FIGURE 1.10 A, B.   Cardiac and pulmonary anatomy.
Adapted from Goldberg S, Ouellette H. *Clinical Anatomy Made Ridiculously Simple.* 3rd ed. Miami, FL: MedMaster; 2007.

TABLE 1.8.   Lung Sounds

Condition	Lung Sounds	Percussion	Fremitus	Egophony
Consolidation	Rales, bronchial	Dull	Increased	Yes
Effusion	Decreased	Dull	Decreased	No
Pneumothorax	Decreased	Tympanitic	Decreased	No
Bronchospasm	Wheeze	Tympanitic	Normal	No

ORTHO EXAM: HAND AND ARM PERIPHERAL NERVES

TABLE 1.9.   Hand and Arm Peripheral Nerves

Nerve	Motor	Sensory	Associated Insult
Radian	Arm extensors	1st dorsal web space	Humeral shaft
Ulnar	Hand intrinsics	4th and 5th finger pad	Elbow
Median	Finger flexors	1st, 2nd, and 3rd finger pad	Wrist
Musculocutaneous	Elbow flexors	Dorsal forearm; radial side	
Axillary	Deltoid	Lateral shoulder/C5	Shoulder, humerus
Suprascapular	Supra- and infraspinatus	N/A	Suprascapular notch

Source: Pregerson DB. *Quick Essentials Emergency Medicine 4.0.* ERPocketbooks.com; 2010:23.

TWO-POINT DISCRIMINATION

■ **Normal:** < 5 mm
■ **Borderline:** 5–10 mm
■ **Abnormal:** > 10 mm

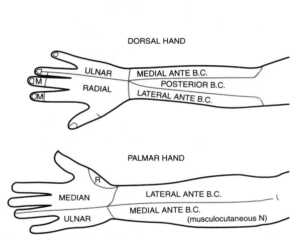

ANTE: ANTERIOR
B.C.: BRACHIAL CUTANEOUS
M: MEDIAN
R: RADIAL
N: NERVE

FIGURE 1.11.   Sensory nerves of the dorsal and palmar hand.

ORTHO EXAM: LEG AND FOOT PERIPHERAL NERVES

TABLE 1.10.   Leg and Foot Peripheral Nerves

Nerve	Motor	Sensory	Associated Insult
Sciatic	Knee flexors	Lower leg	Hip dislocation
Obturator	Hip adductors	Medial thigh	Intrapelvic, symphisis pubis
Femoral	Quadriceps	Anterior thigh	Diabetes mellitus
Posterior tibial	Calf, toe flexors	Sole of foot	Deep compartment, tarsal tunnel
Deep peroneal	Foot dorsiflexors	1st dorsal web space	Tib-fib, anterior compartment
Superficial peroneal	Foot eversion	Dorsal foot	Lateral compartment, fibula

Source: Pregerson DB. *Quick Essentials Emergency Medicine 4.0.* ERPocketbooks.com; 2010:23.

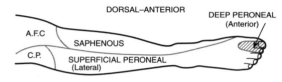

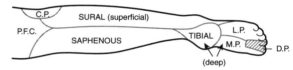

FIGURE 1.12.   Sensory nerves of lower leg (with corresponding compartments in parentheses).

C.P.: Common Peroneal   Anterior Compartment: Deep Peroneal Nerve
D.P.: Deep Peroneal   Deep Posterior Compartment: Tibial and Plantar Nerves
F.C.: Femoral Cutaneous   Lateral Compartment: Superficial Peroneal Nerve
L.P.: Lateral Plantar   Superficial Posterior Compartment: Sural Nerve
M.P.: Medial Plantar

NEURO EXAM

■ Six Parts of the Basic Neuro Exam

- *General*: Orientation, alertness (See Table 1.13)
- *Cranial nerves*: Olfactory, optic, oculomotor, trochlear, trigeminal, abducens, facial, auditory, glossopharyngeal, vagus, spinal accessory, hypoglossal
- *Motor*: Strength scale: 5 = regular, 4 = decreased, 3 = can lift vs. gravity, 2 = motion, 1 = contracts only
- *Sensory*: Pinprick, light touch, temperature, posterior columns (vibration, position)
- *Reflexes*: DTRs, Babinski, special reflexes (see the next section here)
- *Cerebellar*: Romberg, finger-nose-finger, heel shin, tandem gait

TABLE 1.11. Nystagmus

Nystagmus	Latency	Fatigue	Direction	Types	Inhibitors	Enhancers
Peripheral	+/-	Yes	Fixed	→, torsional	Gaze fixing	Gaze to fast phase
Central	No	No	Variable	↑↓, →, torsion	None	Gaze fixation

Source: Pregerson DB. *Quick Essentials Emergency Medicine 4.0.* ERPocketbooks.com; 2010:85.

TABLE 1.12. Glasgow Coma Scale

Points	Eyes	Speech	Motor
1	No response	No response	No response
2	Open to pain	Moans	Extensor posturing to pain
3	Open to command	Words	Flexor posturing to pain
4	Open spontaneously	Confused	Withdraws to pain
5	-----------------------	Oriented x 4	Purposeful; localizes pain
6	-----------------------	-----------------------	Follows complex command

Points for best response: Min = 3, Max = 15.
Coma Terms: Normal level of alertness. Drowsy: Won't keep eyes open (lethargy). Obtunded: Won't open eyes to stimuli/pain. Stuporous: Nonpurposeful response to stimuli/pain.

TABLE 1.13. Mini-Mental Status Exam

Orientation	Year, season, month, date, day	5 points
	Country, state, city, hospital/building, floor	5 points
Memory	Recall three things: short term	3 points
	Recall three things: long term	3 points
Attention	Subtract serial sevens five times OR spell "WORLD" backwards	5 points
Language	Naming (pen and watch) + three-part command: "take R, fold, on floor"	5 points
	Repeat phrase, write sentence, draw pentagons, and "close eyes"	4 points
	Total possible	30 points

■ Special Reflexes (Brain and Spine)

- *Corneals*: Touch cornea with wisp of cotton; should cause blink response
- *Calorics*: Elevate head to 30° and slowly infuse 50 ml of ice water; nystagmus
- *Glabelar*: Frontal release sign: Tap forehead with finger and tell patient to keep eyes from blinking
- *Palmomental*: Frontal release sign: pressing into thumb causes lips to move
- *Cremasteric*: L1 level: Scraping or pressing on inner thigh causes scrotum to contract
- *Bulbocavernosus*: S4 level: Bulbocavernosus: Squeezing penis causes anal sphincter to contract

TABLE 1.14.   NIH Stroke Scale

Topic	NIH Stroke Scale Points	Max Pts.
LOC, general	Alert–0; Drowsy–1; Stuporous–2; Coma–3	3
LOC, questions	Answers both–0; Answers one–1; Wrong on both–2	2
LOC, commands	Obeys both–0; Obeys one–1; Can't obey–2	2
Pupils, reaction	Both react–0; One reacts–1; Neither react–3	3
Gaze, best	Normal–0; Partial palsy–1; Forced deviation–2	2
Vision	No loss–0; Partial hemianopsia–1; Complete hemianopsia–3	3
Facial palsy	Normal–0; Minor–1; Partial–2; Complete–3	3
Arm strength	No drift–0; Drift–1; Can't resist gravity–3; No effort noted–4	4
Leg strength	No drift–0; Drift–1; Can't resist gravity–3; No effort noted–4	4
Babinski	Normal–0; Equivocal–1; Extensor–2; Bilateral extensor–4	4
Limb ataxia	None–0; Upper or lower–1; Upper AND lower–2	2
Sensory	Normal–0; Partial loss–1; Dense loss–2	2
Neglect	None–0; Partial–1; Complete–2	2
Dysarthria	Normal–0; Mild to moderate–1; Near unintelligible–2	2
Aphasia	None–0; Mild to moderate–2; Severe–3; Mute–4	4
	TOTAL POSSIBLE	42

■ **The Spinal Cord**

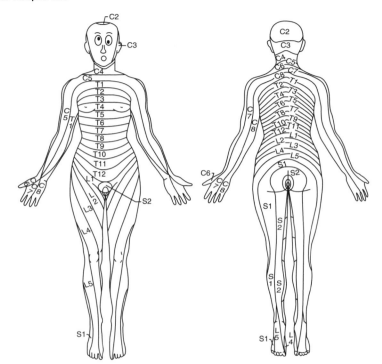

CERVICO-THORACIC SPINAL LEVELS

LEVEL	MOTOR	SENSORY	REFLEX
C3	Trapezius	Occiput	
C4	Diaphragm	Shoulder top	
C5	Biceps, Deltoid	Arm	Biceps
C6	Wrist Extension	Thumb	Biceps
C7	Tricep	Index Finger	Triceps
C8	Finger Flexors	Pinky	Triceps
T1	Interossei	Arm	
T2-T12	Intercotals/Abs	T10 = navel	

LUMBO-SACRAL SPINAL LEVELS

LEVEL	MOTOR	SENSORY	REFLEX
L1	Iliopsoas	Groin crease	Cremaster
L2	Iliopsoas	Leg	
L3	Quads	Medial Thigh	Knee
L4	Quads	Medial Thigh	Knee
L5	EHL	Lateral Calf	
S1	Calf	Outer Foot	Ankle
S2-S4	Rectal sphincter	Perianal, Saddle	Bulbocav

FIGURE 1.13. The neuro exam: The spinal cord.

SECTION 2 ■ DIAGNOSTIC TESTS: EKGs, LAB, AND IMAGING

TESTS: UTILITY, COST, RISKS, AND ADJUSTMENTS

GENERAL WISDOM
- **Names**: Check names on X-rays, labs, etc.
- **Pitfalls**: False negative values are the pitfall of the ill. False positive values are the pitfall of the well.
- **Red Flags**: Address all or consult.
- **Incidentaloma**: Some will be malignant. Always ask radiology if any noted. Always tell patient and PMD. Always check OFFICIAL radiologist ready as the prelim may not note all findings.
- **EKG**: Don't miss old EKG or subtle changes.

CHARGES (NOT COSTS): HOSPITAL/COMMUNITY LABS

EKG and Imaging
EKG: $80–$160
US/Duplex: $600
X-rays: $100 per view
CT scans: $1000–2000
VQ scan: $1000
E-Beam CT: $1500
MRI: $2000
Sestamibi: $1250
HIDA scan: $1250

Blood Work
CBC with dif: $300/$50
Sed Rate: $150/$35
Chem7: $350/$65
LFTs: $300/$60
Amylase: $220/$45
Lipase: $240/$55
Beta HCG: $300/$45
Troponin: $100/$20
BNP: $130/$80
D-dimer: $300/$70
PT: $40/$25
PTT: $40/$25

Micro and Cultures
Urinalysis: $45/$20
Influenza: $50/$25
Pertussis: $45/$25
Rapid strep: $80/$40
RSV: $50/$25
Urine Cx: $380+/$55+
Blood Cx: $380+/$65+
Stool Cx: $360+/$65+
Wound Cx: $340+/$80+
Resp. Cx: $330+/$45+
Throat Cx: $170+/$42+
+ = ↑ price if positive

RISKS OF TESTS
Risks are real.
- **Radiation**: Risk of fatal cancer may be up to 1 in 1000 for certain nuclear scans and CTs. Chest CT = 350 CXRs; Abdo CT = 500 CXRs (see X-rays section on pages 47–52)
- **Contrast**: Risk of kidney damage and anaphylaxis
- **False Positives**: Patient may experience unnecessary anxiety and risks of unnecessary additional testing. Medical treatment predicated on spurious lab results may cause damage.
- **False Negatives**: May miss diagnosis if negative test trusted although suspicion is high
- **Invasive**: Risk of causing a UTI may be up to 1% for an in-and-out cath and higher for a Foley

LAB ADJUSTMENTS
- **Chemistry**: ↑glu100 → ↓Na 1.6; K: Hemolysis can ↑by 2; ↑acetone 100 → ↑Creatinine 1
- **pH**: ↓pH 0.1 → ↑K 0.5; ↑pH 0.1 →↓free Ca 2–8%; ↓bicarb10 →↓pH 0.15; ↑ pCO2 10 →↓pH 0.08(acute) and 0.03 (chronic)
- **Albumin**: ↓Albumin 1 → ↓Ca0.8; Albumin: If = 3, add 3 to gap. If albumin = 2, add 6
  - *Meds*: Dilantin: Measured/(0.9xalbumin/4.4) b/c 90% bound

EKG

BASICS
Other EKGs: R sided (label it), posterior (V7, 8, 9), one interspace lower (COPD)
- **Rhythm**: Wide => three boxes, regular? P wave?; rate (nl RR: 3–5 boxes), blocks, PR interval
- **V Leads**: R > S in V1? R progression, Q?, ST↑, V6 Q-wave = post-MI, LVH; biphasic P: V1, V2
- **Inferior**: ST↑ even < 1 mm is worrisome, P pulmonale ("2 lungs"); Q-wave in III OK if age < 40
- **Lateral**: 1 and aVL: axis, P mitrale ("1 bishop"), LVH if > 11 mm
- **Right**: aVR, V4R: PR elevation?, TCAD (wide QRS)?, R axis; ST↑ in aVR: left main CAD, PE

ARTIFACTS
- **Causes**: Tremor, motion, asterixis, myoclonus, pacer, TENS unit, hiccups, electrical interference
- **Minimizing**: Remove wristwatch, warm blankets, sit on hands
- **Artifacts**: If P-waves and QRS-waves march through then a finding is artifact

NORMAL VARIANTS
- **S1S2S3**: (RVH/PE?); V1: RSR', R = S: 4%; aVL: neg P, QS, neg T
- **RSR'**: Or incomplete right bundle branch block
- **Obese**: Decreased amplitude, flatter or T-waves in 2, 3, AVF. Flat or inverted Ts in lateral leads, LVH
- **Pregnant**: S1Q3T3; T inversion and ST depress in limb and V1–2; LAD, Q inferior
- **Age < 40**: Q in III OK if age < 40; bad R progress age < 40; V1 inverted T = "persistent juvenile"
- **Peds**: PR: 90–140; RV > LV up to 6 mon; max HR = 170–10 (age in yr); Q: Lateral, inferior; T should be down in V1 from 7d–7 yr, but may persist

THE 4 PS: PERICARDITIS, PULMONARY EMBOLISM, PNEUMOTHORAX, POTASSIUM
- **Pericarditis**: Diffuse ST↑ (except in R, V1, III, L), PR depression, T-wave flattening/depression
  - *Other*: Abnl P-wave, A-fib/flutter

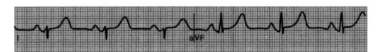

FIGURE 2.1. Pericarditis.

  - *Effusion*: Low voltage, alternans, tachycardia
  - *vs MI*: Likely pericarditis: concave up, no reciprocal Δ's, diffuse Δ's, no Q-wave; ST↑ in II>III.
    Likely pericarditis: Best is V6 ST:T ratio: if ST↑ height/Twave height > 0.24 in V6.
    Likely AMI if: ST↑ convex up or greater in lead III than II, reciprocal Δ's, new Q's.
  - Stage 1: ST elevation; Stage 2: ST nl, flat T; Stage 3: T inversion; Stage 4: All back to Normal
- **PE**: RV dilate > clockwise = S1Q3 + RBBB. If ischemia get ST&T changes or atrial dysr/AVB; RAD, transient, flip T V1–V4, LAD; QR, R > S or R > 5 mm in V1, ST ↑↓(esp. aVR), P pulmonale; EKG can mimic: MI (inferior, anterior), pulmonary disease; can be WNL, IRBBB, transient BBB
- **P = coPd**: P: P pulmonale II and III, tall P inferior > 2.5 mm, P axis > 80°; Q anterior, poor R progression, low amplitude, esp. I, deep S inferior + lateral, RAD, clockwise
- **Pneumothorax**: Low voltage, MI mimic (Q, ST up, flip T), RAD, ST↑ V1–4
- **Potassium**: See Electrolytes section on page 28

WAVES AND INTERVALS

- **P Wave:** P PR: Short PR: WPW, low Ca, Lown-Ganong-Levine, (ASD)
  - *Long PR*: ↑Ca
  - *P-axis*: Normal 0–75°: Up in I, down in R, biphasic in V1. Inverted: Ectopic pacer.
  - *Big RA*: Right atrial enlargement: amplitude > 2.5 boxes; DDx: ASD, PHTN, Pulm dz
  - *Big LA*: Left atrial enlargement: wide P-wave > 0.11 sec; DDx: MS, MR, LVH, AI, AR
- **QRS Axis:** WNL: 0–105°, age > 40: -30–90°; q in III OK age < 40; depolarization: septal > free wall > basal

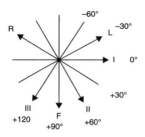

FIGURE 2.2.   QRS axis.
Reproduced with permission from Argyle B. MicroEKG Computer Program Manual. Mad Scientist Software, Alpine, Utah.

- - *RAD*: Normal variant: Low diaphragm, tall and thin, children; RBBB, LPFB, pacer, dextrocardia, PE, RVH, PHTN, WPW, VT, COPD, ASD, VSD
  - *LAD*: Normal, LVH, PE, LBBB, LAHB, WPW, ↑QRS, ↑K, COPD, tricuspid atresia
- **QRS Wide:** WPW, BBB, IVCD, LVH; ↑K, ↑Ca, cold; VT, PE, CM, carditis. Drugs: Class 1B and C, dig, BB, CCB, TCA
  - *LBBB*: Criteria: QRS > 0.12, lead 1 upright with slur/notch, leads V4, V5, or V6 with RSR', 2° ST–TΔs. Cxs: "CHARCOAL" (**C**AD : 80% > **H**TN > **A**S, **R**HD, **C**M, **O**ther, **L**ev's); meds: BB, TCA, dig
  - *RBBB*: Criteria: QRS > 0.12, lead 1 biphasic and broad S, leads V1, V2, or V3 with RSR', 2° ST–TΔs. Cxs: CAD: 5% AMI > HTN, RHD, cor pulm: 9% PE, carditis, degen, trauma/surgery, congen, NL, ↑K
  - *RSR' V1*: NL (V1R < 8 mm + R' < 6 + R'/s < 1), RVH (R' > 10–15 + abnl P). Cxs: Incomplete RBBB, PE, true post-MI: T-wave likely UPRIGHT, skeletal, leads, Brugada
  - *LPFB*: Rare. Criteria: Axis 90–180, S1Q3 and no other cause of RAD, no RVH, small q in II, III, aVF. Cxs: CAD > HTN, CM, AV, dissection
  - *LAFB*: Axis < -45°, small q's leads I and aVL, small r's leads II, III, and aVF. rS inferior + LAD; = LAD ŝLVH. Cxs: CAD: 34% > HTN: 14% > AMI: 4% > AV valve, CM, degenerative, ↑K
- **QRS Voltage:** Alternans: CAD, rheumatic heart disease, cor pulmonale, pericarditis/tamponade, WPW
  - *LVH*: Criteria: any of aVL > 11 mm, I > 15 mm, V5 > 30 mm, S in V1 + R in V5 or V6 ≥ 35 mm, others
  - *Low volt*: All limb R + S < 5: PTX, effuse (CHF, thyroid, pericarditis, CABG), COPD, amyloid, scar, scleroderma
- **Q-Wave:** Normal "septal Q": < 0.03 sec, < 4 mm or 25% QRS (in III 0.04 sec and 5 mm [1 box x 5 box])
- **S-Wave:** < 3 mm in V1 = RVH, post-MI (intrinsicoid deflection = Q to R peak)
- **ST-Normal:** 1–3 mm↑ in V1–V4:91% (most at V2, only 20% women); MI can be concave up!
  - *BER*: Age < 50, T > 4x ST, V2–V5, no reciprocal Δ, stable, notched/hook, concave up, < 3 mm
  - *ST↑*: BER, RBBB, LBBB, LVH, MI, PE (esp. AVR), ↑K, pericarditis, pacer, LV aneurysm, ↑Ca+, Brugada, ST↑ in lead aVR: PE, L-main CAD disease
  - *ST↓*: Ischemia (flat, upsloping), reciprocal Δ: (inferior > anterior), BBB, LVH, dig., WPW, MVP, ↑K
- **J-Point↑:** DDx: Early repol., ↑calcemia, Brugada, hypothermia, MI, pericarditis, LVH, myocarditis, ↑K

■ **T-Wave:** Cardiac repolarization; normal amplitude < 5 boxes limb leads and 10 boxes precordial
  ● *T-V1:* A large upright T-wave in V1 is suggestive of acute ischemia, especially if it is new.
  ● *NSTWC:* "ESCAPED" (**E**lectrolyte, **S**tress, **C**ardiac, **A**bdo, **P**E/pericarditis, **E**ndocrine, **D**rug)
  ● *Peak T:* (Computer will not pick this up): DDx: MI, LBBB, RBBB, pacer, LVH, BER, pericarditis, hemopericar-dium, valvular dz, IHSS; ↑K (narrow and symmetric), hyperthyroid, anemia, ↑Mg

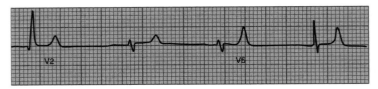

FIGURE 2.3.   Peaked T-wave.

  ● *Flat T:* ↓K, ↓Ca, ↓Mg, pericarditis, digoxin, psych meds, ischemia, heart disease
  ● *Biphasic:* ACS, nl, Wellen's (See Ischemia section on pages 21–22)
  ● *Invert T:* Danger: ACS, Wellen's (biphasic): LAD lesion, myocarditis, MI, PE, CNS, BBB, WPW. Coronary T-wave: Flip T preceded by near isoelectric convex up ST. Others: Juvenile (ant flip T), LVH, Digoxin, hyperventilation, post meal, nl variant. LVH T-wave (depressed J, asymmetric/hockey stick, terminal positivity, V6 > V4); limb lead reversal, pericarditis, persistent juvenile pattern, paced, past MI.
■ **QT Long:** EKG computer may use 440–450, but 10–20% of normal population has QTc longer than that. Ninety-ninth percentile for normal is QTc > 470 in men and QTc > 480 in women. QTc > 500 dangerous.

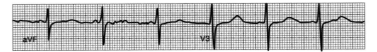

FIGURE 2.4.   Long QT.

  ● *Risk:* Higher if female, multiple factors, coronary disease
  ● *Disease:* CAD, MVP, cardiomyopathy, CVA, SAH, Lange-Nielsen (deafness), Romano-Ward
  ● *Lytes:* ↓K, ↓Ca, ↓Mg, ↓phosphorus
  ● *Tox:* Arsenic, coke, organophosphates, methadone, ↑lithium
  ● *Meds:* Heart: Amiodarone, sotalol, ibutilide, procainamide, quinidine. ABX: Biaxin, -azole drugs, pentamidine, amantidine, Ketek, EES, quinolones. Other: TCA, phenothiazines, cisapride, Tacrolimus, lithium
■ **QT Short:** < 350 msec. DDx: ↑Ca, Dig, ↑K, congenital; can be associated with sudden death too
■ **U-Wave:** Can be normal variant. Abnl if > 1.5 mm or > 25% height of T-wave in any lead
  ● *DDx:* Ischemia, bradycardia, ↓K, ↓Ca, ↑Ca, CNS, LVH, TSH, MVP, pheochromocytoma, exercise
  ● *Meds:* Digoxin, amiodarone, quinidine

ISCHEMIA

Get Serial EKGS

- **Basics**: Always get serial EKGs and old EKG, even if from PMD office or other hospital; ischemia→delay repolarization→ flip/tall T; injury > partial depolarization → ST↑; infarct = silent zone → Q-wave
- **Timing**: Peak T (min-hours) > ST↑ (< 1 mm)(reciprocal in 80%)(h-days)(measure 1 mm from J) > Q (2–14 hr) onset; usually developed by 9 hr; last days; permanent in 85%) (Abnormal Q ≥0.04 sec. Q ≥ 1 box, > 25% except in V1, III, R, and ?L) > T inversion (can be temporary or permanent)
- **Findings**: ST↑:40%, or ST↓:75%, or old MI: 85%, or NSSTWC: 90%, NI: 10% (#1 cause of miss)
- **Pseudo MI**: MI mimics usually are stable over time and are not associated with reciprocal changes. Causes: LVH (ST↑ V1–2, ST↓ V3–6, poor R progress, strain, QS), RVH, COPD (Q, poor R progress), PTX (T↓), PE (ST ↑or↓, T↓) ICH (ST ↑or↓+ large T up or down), hyperkalemia (ST↑ V1V2 ū with short QT); others: LV aneurysm, benign early repolarization, pericarditis
- **Badness**: ST↑ > dynamic Δs > ST↓ (50% from MI) > LBBB > paced > old MI > deep/peak T > LVH
- **Findings**: ST↑:40%, or ST↓:75%, or old MI: 85%, or NSSTWC: 90%, NI: 10% (#1 cause of missed MI)
- **Prinzmental**: Recurrent and transient ST↑ at rest during chest pain w/o ↑Trop
- **Reperfusion**: CP and ST improve/resolve by > 70% in < 30–90 min (If not, need Rescue PTCA). T-wave inversion: < 4 hr. AIVR: 90%, PVC, VT: 20%, bradycardia
- **Normal**: Normal in 10%, even during chest pain; risk of bad outcome still just as high

TABLE 2.1. Classification of Ischemic Changes on EKG by Location

Wall	Artery	EKG Changes and Notes
Anterior	Left anterior descending	ST↑ ≥ 2 mm in V2–V4 Other: Reciprocal depression in II, III, aVF in 33%; new RBBB with Q in V1 Comps: block needing pacer, hypotension, aneurysm
Inferior	Right coronary > circumflex	II, III, and aVF: ST↑ ≥ 0.8–1 mm, but may be minimal, usually lead III > II Reciprocal ST↓ in aVL in 80% and often marked (if none consider other dz) Comps: RVMI in 30%, bradycardia and blocks that are often temporary
Lateral	Circumflex	ST↑ ≥ 1–2 mm in V5–V6 or ST↑ ≥ 1 mm in I, aVL Other: May also cause some anterior, inferior, or posterior wall infarction
Posterior	Right coronary circumflex	V1–V2: tall R or rR', rSR' or ST↓, peaked T V6: Q-wave V8–V9: tall R/T, S < 3, ST↑ ≥ 1mm
RVMI	Right coronary circumflex	ST↑ 1 mm V4R (often also V1 and V2, which is suggestive) ST↓ in aVL: 87%/91% Note: Complicates 30% of inferior MIs and 13% of anterior MIs

■ **Acute Coronary Syndrome: Special Cases**

- *MI and RBBB*: ST segments normally isoelectric except for slight ST depression V1-V3. If ST↑ worry; if acute, should be from large anterior MI.
- *MI and LBBB*: Sgarbossa Criteria: Any of following in LBBB or paced rhythm suggests AMI. If acute, should have ongoing chest pain or other sx.
  1. ST elevation that is appropriately discordant with end of QRS but is > 5 mm: 31%/92%

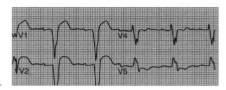

FIGURE 2.5.   Ischemic EKG by the Sgarbossa Criteria.

  2. ST elevation > 1 mm that is inappropriately concordant with end of QRS: 73%/92%

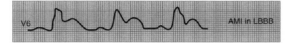

FIGURE 2.6.   Sgarbossa positive by item 2.
Source: Pregerson DB. *Quick Essentials Emergency Medicine 4.0.* ERPocketbooks.com; 2010:56.

  3. ST depression > 1 mm in V1, V2, or V3: 25%/96%
  4. Upright T-wave in V5 or V6: 26%/92%.
  5. Left axis deviation: 72%/48%

- *MI and pacer:* Most pacers in RV so normal pattern is an LBBB; Sgarbossa less accurate, but best is #1. ST elevation that is appropriately discordant with end of QRS but is > 5 mm: 53%/88%
- *Lead AVR*: ST↑ can be RVMI, LAD, or left main disease or PULMONARY EMBOLISM
- *T-V1*: A large upright T-wave in V1 is suggestive of acute ischemia, especially if it is new

FIGURE 2.7.   T-V1 ischemic finding.
Source: Pregerson DB. *Quick Essentials Emergency Medicine 4.0.* ERPocketbooks.com; 2010:56.

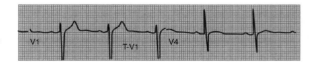

- *Wellen's*: Bad proximal LAD coronary stenosis: biphasic or deep T-waves in V2–V3. Δs usually occur while pain-free and appear nonspecific, but portend a tight proximal LAD lesion. Rx: Do not do a stress test—too risky. Go straight to cath instead.

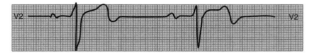

FIGURE 2.8.   Wellen's warning for ischemia on EKG.
Source: Pregerson DB. *Quick Essentials Emergency Medicine 4.0.* ERPocketbooks.com; 2010:56.

EXERCISE STRESS TESTS AND ADVANCED CARDIAC EVALUATION

- ■ **Basics:** 50–70% stenosis is considered a "significant" lesion warranting intervention
  - ● *Utility*: Sensitivity: 50–85%. Specificity: 75–90%. Test performs worse in unselected population
- ■ **Contraindications:** Unstable angina, symptomatic CHF, symptomatic or severe aortic stenosis, acute PE. Evolving EKG changes, elevated troponin, BP >200/110, angiography indicated. MI within 2 days, uncontrolled arrhythmia, pericarditis, myocarditis, aortic dissection
  - ● *Relative*: Left main disease, moderate valvular disease, electrolyte abnormality, hypoxia, beta blocker. Inability to exercise, AV-block, bundle branch block, hypertrophic cardiomyopathy, arrhythmia
- ■ **Preparation:** NPO for at least 2 hours. No caffeine x 24h before nuclear medicine studies
- ■ **Stop Test:** Symptoms (ataxia, weak, angina…), ST↓ of 2 mm, Systolic BP↓10 mmHg, pallor, DBP > 115. Patient desire to stop, arrhythmia, QRS becomes wide, ST↑ > 1 mm in leads without Q-waves
- ■ **Adequacy:** Did they walk long enough? What was the peak heart rate? During test BP – HR should ↑. Inconclusive if don't reach 10 METs of 85% of max predicted heart rate (max HR = 220 − age).
- ■ **Positive:** Flat or downsloping ST↓ of 1 mm for >2 boxes that was not pre-existing.
- ■ **MET's:** Metabolic Equivalents: gives good prognostic info regardless of the rest of the test. 1: rest. 2: walking at 2 mph. 4: walking at 4 mph. 5: peak for activities of daily living. 10: prognosis with medical rx as good as bypass. 13: excellent prognosis. 18: Elite athlete
- ■ **Poor Man's:** Dr. Slovis recommends considering the following on a low risk patient you plan to send home: Have pt. run in place until HR >75% max, then do an EKG. If ST changes or pain, admit.
- ■ **Sestamibi:** 85–90%/70–85%. Time between rest and stress images = 4h. (See Nuclear Medicine Tests section on page 65). Higher sensitivity for other tests, especially for single vessel disease of left circumflex. Best prognostic information due to larger databases
- ■ **Adenosine:** Use if patient cannot exercise or has an AICD. Contraindicated if caffeine intake past 12–24h. Avoid in patients with asthma/COPD or bradyarrhythmias
- ■ **Stress Echo:** 85%/81%. Image quality adversely affected by obesity or COPD. No radiation. More specific but less sensitive than sestamibi. Valve and functional assessment
- ■ **Dobutamine:** Can precipitate arrhythmia and death in 1 of 5000, so MD should be present

TABLE 2.2   Pre-test Likelihood of Coronary Disease

Age	Non-Anginal Pain		Atypical Pain		Typical Angina	
2 years	Men	Women	Men	Women	Men	Women
35	3–35	1–19	8–59	2–39	30–68	10–78
45	9–47	2–22	21–70	5–43	51–92	20–79
55	23–59	4–25	45–79	10–47	80–95	38–82
65	40–69	9–29	71–86	20–51	93–97	56–84

Lower number for patient without cardiac risk factors; higher number is if all cardiac risk factors present

BRADYCARDIA

- **DDx**
  - *Low*: O_2, glucose, temperature
  - *High*: K, Trop, TSH
  - *Tox*: Amiodarone, BB, CCB, Dig, clonidine, lithium
  - *Cardiac*: Degenerative, ischemic, sick-sinus, postoperative, traumatic, post-ID
- **1° AV Block**: PR > 200: Vagal, degen., ischemia, drugs (dig, IA, CCB/BB), carditis (ARF, Chaga's, Lyme, dT)
- **2° AV Block**: Two types: Mobitz 1and Mobitz 2
  - *Mobitz 1*: Gradual prolonging of PR interval before dropped QRS: usually not infranodal; DDx: Vagal, degen, ischemia, drugs (dig, IA, CCB/BB), carditis (ARF, Chaga, Lyme, dT), AR
  - *Mobitz 2*: Dropped QRS without preceding prolongation of PR interval. Often infranodal. DDx: Degenerative, anterior MI, calcific AS; if QRS wide in Mobitz 1 treat as Mobitz 2

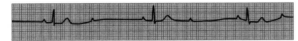

FIGURE 2.9.   Second degree AV block, Mobitz type 2.
Source: Pregerson DB. *Quick Essentials Emergency Medicine 4.0*. ERPocketbooks.com; 2010:59.

- **3° AV Block**: No relationship between P-wave and QRS. QRS usually wide
  DDx: Congenital, post-op/trauma, carditis, Ca↑ or ↓; in AMI atropine can > VT/VF in AVB 2b and 3

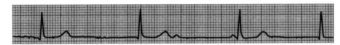

FIGURE 2.10.   Third degree AV block.

- **Hyperkalemia**: K < 7: peak T, S in I/V6, S1Q3T3. K = 7–8: ST↑, wide: P/QRS, AVB, brady K > 8: wide QRS,VF

FIGURE 2.11.   Severe hyperkalemia with sine waves.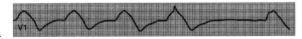

- **Hypothermia**: "BASO" (**B**radycardia, **A**-fib, **S**hiver artifact, **O**sborne J's > ↑ intervals, junctional, Vfib, ST↑)

FIGURE 2.12.   Hypothermia with Osborne J-waves and shiver artifact.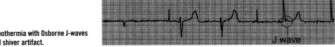

- **Idioventricular Rhythm**: Preterminal rhythm: MI, tamponade, exsanguination
- **Junctional**: No P, flat baseline: ischemia, Dig, K↑, Verapamil, CCB, BB, degenerative

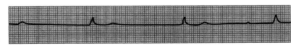

FIGURE 2.13.   Junctional rhythm.

- **Sinus Bradycardia**: Athlete, increased vagal tone, drugs

INFECTIONS

Infections affecting the heart often cause heart block.

■ **Viral**: HIV, rubella
■ **Parasitic**: Chaga's, trichinosis
■ **Bacterial**: Lyme, leptospirosis, diphtheria, tetanus, pertussis, strep, typhoid, mycoplasma

SYNCOPE OR PALPITATIONS

■ **Stigmata:** Any of the findings below should raise concern about life-threatening arrhythmia potential
  • *Bradycardia*: See page 24
  • *Brugada Syndrome:*

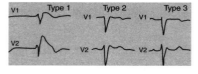

FIGURE 2.14.   Brugada syndrome.
Source: Pregerson DB. *Quick Essentials Emergency Medicine 4.0.*
ERPocketbooks.com; 2010:63.

  Down-sloping ST↑ V1-V3 ūwith neg T wave; 10%/y die w/out AICD; screen family, esp Asian. DDx: ↑K, ↑Ca, drug tox, RV injury, nl variant (no syncope), Brugada (50/50 sporadic/familial)

  • **Hypertrophic Obstructive CardioMyopathy (HOCM)**: Deep narrow Q waves in I, avL, v5, v6
  • **Ischemia**: Q wave, LAFB, BBB, ST changes, T wave changes, etc.
  • **Long QT**: Risks for Torsade: Bradycardia, CHF, MI, female, multiple factors, T-wave alternans. Dx: EKG computer may use 440–450, but 10–20% of normal population has QTc longer than that ninety-ninth percentile for normal is QTc > 470 in men and QTc > 480 in women. QTc > 500 dangerous. Causes: Tox/meds, CAD, K/Mg/Ca/PO4. Congenital: Romano-Ward (can hear) and Jaervell-Lang-Nielson (deaf).

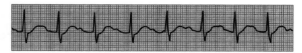

FIGURE 2.15.   Long QT interval.

  • **RV Dysplasia**: Arrhythmogenic RV Dysplasia - big RA; RV electrically silent as is all scar and fat. Get V-tach

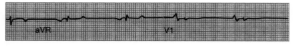

FIGURE 2.16.   Right ventricular dysplasia.

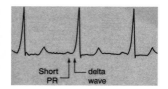

FIGURE 2.17.   Wolff-Parkinson-White.
Source: Pregerson DB. *Quick Essentials Emergency Medicine 4.0.*
EMresource.org; 2010:63.

  • **Short PR**: Wolff-Parkinson-White: Short PR +/- delta wave. Lown Ganong Levine: Short PR and no delta wave. Hypocalcemia: Short PR with long QT.
  • **Tachycardia:** See pages 26–27

TACHYCARDIAS: NARROW

- ■ **Narrow**: Look for P-wave (if strange P, compare it to prior EKG)
- ■ **Regular**: PSVT, flutter
- ■ **Irregular**: A-fib, MAT, flutter, PAT with variable block, sinus with PACs, flutter with variable block; wandering pacemaker, sinus arrhythmia, 2nd-degree block, NSR with sinus pause
- ■ **Atrial Ectopic Tachycardia (AET)**: HR > 100 (120–250), short PR

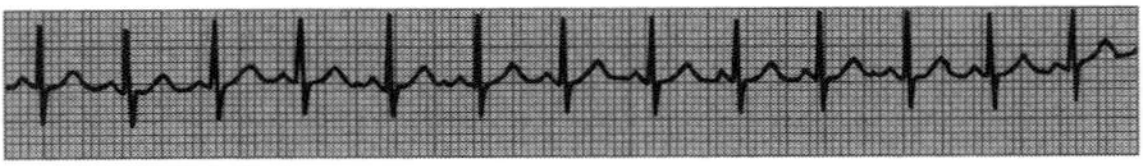

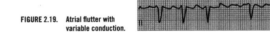

FIGURE 2.18. Atrial ectopic tachycardia.

- ● *DDx/Rx*: COPD, dig toxic, re-entry, ↑ automaticity; Rx: Often refractory, nodal blockers don't work
- ■ **Atrial Fibrillation**
  - ● *Worry*: They are sick! Atrial kick = 15% EF. Rates: 110–140: New or Ppt. Slow: Block, med, SSS. > 150: Ppt: Often pain, ID. > 200: WPW?. Ppt: Anything to ↑ sympathetic drive: pain, drug or withdrawal, sepsis, TSH, MI, dehydration
- ■ **Atrial Flutter:** 150 (125–170); DDx: MI, TSH, PE, mitral valve, surgery, COPD, CAD, ↓Mg, ↓K

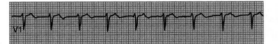

FIGURE 2.19. Atrial flutter with variable conduction.

- ■ **Junctional**: Narrow at 70–130 bpm, PR < 120, P' wave.
  - ● *Causes*: ↑K, Dig > MI, carditis
  - ● *Rx*: Don't shock, electricity doesn't work. Treat primary cause. Can try overdrive pacing.

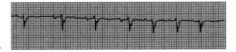

FIGURE 2.20. Junctional tachycardia.

- ■ **Multifocal Atrial Tachycardia (MAT)**: HR > 100 with multiple different P-waves
  - ● *Causes*: Dig. toxic, Mg, K, COPD, sepsis, CHF, theophyline, hypoxia

FIGURE 2.21. Multifocal atrial tachycardia.

- ■ **Sick Sinus Syndrome**: Careful with CCB or BB as may brady down
- ■ **Supra-Ventricular Tachycardia (SVT)**: Rate 125–250 and regular; if > 200: consider WPW
  - ● *Causes*: "TWAM" (TCAD, WPW, ASD, MI, MVP). Labs: Trop, electrolytes

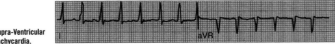

FIGURE 2.22. Supra-Ventricular Tachycardia.

TACHYCARDIAS: WIDE

■ **Irregular**: A-fib with bundle branch block, WPW (esp. if HR > 200), torsade, polymorphic VT

■ **Regular**: VT, ↑K, ischemia, recent cardioversion, meds (procainamide, flecanide, TCAs) (WPW is so fast it may look regular)

■ **Premature Ventricular Contractions (PVCs)**: Compensatory pause; occasionally narrow, multifocal or fusion?
  ● *DDx*: CAD, MI, dig, low K/Mg/O₂, hi Ca, alkalosis, MVP, drugs (procainamide, psych meds), benign
  ● *Grades*: 1: < 30/hr; 2: > 30/hr; 3: multifocal; 4: A: couplets, B: salvos of three; 5: R on T
  ● *Rx*: K to keep K > 4, Mg, beta blocker (NOT if sustained V-Tach, consult if unsure). Lidocaine: consider for: multifocal PVCs, R on T, nonsustained VT (< 30 sec, BP ok). Class III for PVCs (↑asystole), AIVR; not usually used for couplets

■ **Accelerated Idio-Ventricular Rhythm (AIVR)**: Rate < 120. Causes: AMI, reperfusion, digoxin
  ● *Rx*: Benign, don't treat it. Giving lidocaine could cause asystole.

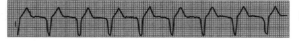

FIGURE 2.23. Accelerated idio-ventricular rhythm.

■ **Ventricular Tachycardia (V-Tach)**: Rate 120–200, regular, wide. PVCs, 3°AVB, QRS > 140, extreme LAD, concordant QRSs; sustained = > 30 sec or BP↓; capture/fusion beats. Adenosine sensitive V-tach: admit ICU

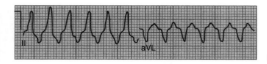

FIGURE 2.24. Ventricular tachycardia.

  ● *DDx*: SVT with aberrancy, WPW, AIVR (rate usually < 120), hyperkalemia (rate usually < 120)
  ● *Cx*: "ABCs": **A**ir (O₂), **B**lood (ACS, Hb, BP), **C**atechol, **D**rug (coke, TCA, opiate, dig), **E**lectrolytes (K, Mg); also: CM, valve, drugs (pentamidine, EtOH, hydrocarbons), trauma, long QT, sarcoid

■ **Torsade**: Polymorphic V-tach, rate 150–300, irregular. Usually self terminates but may → V-fib.

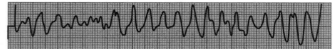

FIGURE 2.25. Torsade-de-pointes.

  ● *Causes*: See Long QT
  ● *RF*: ↑Age, female, CHF, bradycardia
  ● *Rx*: Mg up to 10 g, 200 J. Prevent recurrence with isuprel or pacing at 90–120. NO: amiodarone or procainamide because both prolong the QT interval

■ **Wide SVT**: Only surefire Dx is to have an old EKG. Brugada himself missed 2%. Assume V-tach.

■ **WPW**: Wide and irregular, bizarre (mimics V-tach), rate > 200 → V-fib. Rx: cardiovert, procainamide

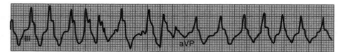

FIGURE 2.26. Wolff-Parkinson-White syndrome (WPW).

ELECTROLYTES

- **K-High**: K < 7: peak T-wave, BER, S-wave in I or V6, S1Q3T3: compare to old EKG.
- **K = 7–8**: ST elevation, wide: P/QRS, AV block, bradycardia, RBBB K > 8: wide QRS, V-fib

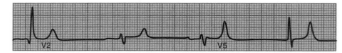

FIGURE 2.27.   Hyperkalemia: Peaked T-waves.

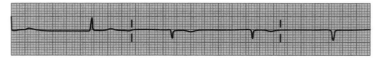

FIGURE 2.28.   Hyperkalemia: Junctional rhythm.

- **K-Low**: K > 2.6: U-wave, flat T-wave, (U > T in V2 + V3); K < 2.6: ST depression > Himalayan T-waves > wide QRS

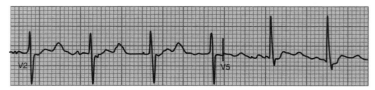

FIGURE 2.29.   Hypokalemia: Large U-wave.

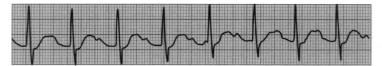

FIGURE 2.30.   Himalayan T-waves.

- **Ca-High**: Short ST and short QT (QTc less than 350), long PR and long QRS
- **Ca-Low**: Long QT often with normal T and long ST, short PR and short QRS, > flat or inverted T
- **Mg-High**: Short PR, peak T-wave, wide QRS, AV blocks
- **Mg-Low**: Long QT usually with flat T-wave, A-fib, ventricular and supraventricular dysrhythmias

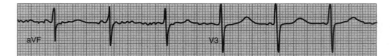

FIGURE 2.31.   Hypomagnesemia: QT prolongation.

DRUGS

- **Amiodarone**: Long QT, bradycardia (beta-blocking action)
- **Digoxin**: Short QT, flip/flat T, ST depress, anything; Tox = "PB&J" (**P**VC > V-tach, **B**rady > block, **J**xnl)

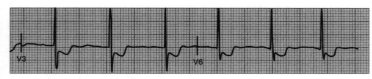

FIGURE 2.32. ST depression from toxic digoxin level.

- **Psych Meds**: Therapeutic: 50% have U, flat or invert T, ST depress, long QT (mimic hypoK)
  - *Toxic*: ↑HR, ↑QT, QRS > 100, conduction delays, ↑automaticity, ventricular dysrhythmias

LAB

BASICS
- **Bell Curve**: Of normal people, 2.5% will have values slightly high and 2.5% will have values slightly low.
- **False -/+'s**: Do not trust normal results in an ill patient or abnormal results in a well patient.
- **Beware**: Beware of treating spurious lab results (no Sx or Sn, nl EKG)
- **Repeat**: GI bleed: CBC q4h x 3; DKA: BMP q1–2h until improving then q4
- **Stat**: Some ER labs can get a 2-min turnaround on whole blood in a green top
- **Altered**: "TACOMA" (Trop, Tox, Ammonia, CO_2, CO, Ca, O_2, Osmolality, Mg, Alcohol)
- **↓Anion Gap**: Low Na, low albumin, bromine (HBr in many meds), iodine, lithium, multiple myeloma
- **↑Anion Gap**: "MUD PILES" (Methanol, Uremia, DKA, Paraldehyde, INH, iron Lactate, Ethanol, Salicylates)

TABLE 2.3.   Collecting Specimens

Tube Color	Inversions	Additives	Tests
Light blue	4	Na-Citrate	PT, PTT, D-dimer, fibrinogen
Green	10	Heparin	Troponin, ammonia, free calcium
Grey	10	Na-Fluoride	Lactic acid
Purple or pink	10	EDTA	CBC, B-natiuritic peptide, HBA1C, Kleihaur-Betke
Red	5	Nothing	Chemistry, tox, LFTs, amylase/lipase, blood bank, ESR
Tiger	10	Separator	Most, but not all of studies for red top
Cultures	10	Broth	Blood cultures

FORMULAE
For more information, go to www.mdcalc.com
- **Aa gradient**: Aa = 150 - pO_2 - (1.25) pCO_2 (at sea level on room air). nl = 5–15
- **Adjustments**: ↑glucose of 100 → ↓Na of 1.6 pH↓ by 0.1 → ↑K by 0.6; hemolysis can ↑K by 2; ↓Albumin of 1 → ↓Ca of 0.8; pH↑ by 0.1 → ↓Ca by 0.12; ↑acetone 100 → ↑Cr 1
- **Anion Gap**: Na–(Cl+ HCO_3) [normal = 7–16] Albumin and anion gap: If = 3, add 3 to gap. If = 2, add 6 to gap.
- **EtOH**: Metabolized at a rate of about 25/hr or some say 10–20/hr (up to 25–35 in chronic alcoholics)
- **FENa**: (Urine Na/plasma Na)/(urine creatinine/plasma creatinine) x 100
- **GFR**: AKA Cr clearance: (lean kg)(140 - age)(0.85 if female)/(72)(stable creatinine); nl: > 80
- **Osmolality**: 2(Na) + glucose/18 + BUN/2.8 + ethanol/4.6 + methanol/3.2 + isopropanol/6.4 (nl 290–300)
- **Osmolal Gap**: Measured osmolality (normal: 280–300) – Calculated osmolality
  - *DDx*: Isopropanol/6 + methanol/3.2 + ethylene-glycol/6.2, error, timing difference in blood draws

MY LAB RECORDS
- **ABGs**: pH: 6.66, 7.66; pCO_2: 141, 9
- **Cardiac**: CK: 648,000; troponin: 777
- **CBC**: Hb: 3.4; platelets: 8; bands: 60
- **Chemistry**: Na: 97,183; K: 9.7, 1.1; Ca: 17.3; Mg: 0.2; bicarb: 4, 65; BUN: 321; glucose: 2003
- **LFTs/GI**: Bilirubin: 30; lipase: 40,000
- **Tox**: EtOH: 628; INR: 45

ELECTROLYTES

Critical values: K: 2.5/6.0; Na: 125/150; Ca: 6/13; Mg: 1.0/3.0; P: 1.0

- **Calcium↑**: DDx (all may ↓ PO_4): CA, MM, PTH, endocrine, ID, Li, HCTZ, Addison, thyrotox, pheo, Paget's
  - *Sx/EKG*: Dehydration, polyuria, stones, groans, psych
  - *EKG*: Brady, AVB, BBB
- **Calcium↓**: DDx: CA, ID, ↓PTH, pancreatitis, rhabdo, alkalosis, meds
  - *Sx/EKG*: CHF, ↓BP, psych; ↑DTR, tetany, Chvostek, sz
  - *EKG*: Short PR, long ST/QT > flat/invert T
  - *Check*: Ionized Ca (normal is 4.5–5.6), albumin, Mg, PO_4
- **Magnesium↑**: DDx: ESRD/ARF, iatrogenic, meds (Mylanta, MOM)
  - *Sx/EKG*: Tingle, low BP, AMS, (8: lose DTR, 12: arrest)
  - *EKG*: Short PR, peak T, ↑QRS, block
- **Magnesium↓**: DDx: Diuretic, diarrhea, malnutrition, ↑Ca++, Conn's
  - *Sx/EKG*: Weak, DTR↑, tremor, tetany, Sz, AMS, N/V
  - *EKG*: Long QT/PR, flat T, Afib, Torsade
- **Phosphorus↑**: ESRD, laxative, PTH, acidosis, rhabdo
  - *Rx*: Keep Ca x PO_4 < 70; $CaCO_3$, insulin + glu, HD
- **Phosphorus↓**
  - *DDx*: Malabsorption, antacid, renal, shift
  - *Rx*: Neutraphos, phos < 1: give IV
  - *Sx/EKG*: Weak, sz, coma, rhabdo
  - *EKG*: Long QT
- **Potassium↑**
  - *DDx*: "BAD STAR" (**B**B, **A**CEI, **A**ldactone, **D**ig, **S**eptra, **T**PN, **A**ddison, **A**cid, **R**enal, **R**habdo)
  - *Sx/EKG*: Weakness. K > 6: admit telemetry; EKG: Peak T, RBBB, wide QRS
- **Potassium↓**
  - *DDx*: Shift: catecols, meds; GU: Lasix, steroids, RTA, ↓Mg, ↓Ca, Barters; GI: V/D, laxative
  - *Sx/EKG*: Weak, constipation; check magnesium level; EKG: flat T > ↓ST > U > ↑QRS > V-fib
- **Sodium↑**
  - *DDx*: Dehyd, DI (UA sg < 1.005); CNS: pituitary, trauma
  - *Renal*: Li, cisplatin, sickle, myeloma
  - *Sx/Tests*: Thirst, N/V, AMS; check: Osm, UNa; if Na > 160/sx: ICU, and consider CT (bleed, thrombosis)
- **Sodium↓**
  - *DDx hypovolemic*: GU: lasix, meds; GI: V, D
  - *DDx hypervolemic*: CHF, ESLD, ESRD
  - *DDx normovolemic*: SIADH
  - *Sx/EKG*: HA, AMS, N, V. Test: Osmolality, UNa
  - *Admit*: < 120, < 125 + comorb/sx

RENAL FUNCTION TESTS AND GLUCOSE, KETONES, LACTATE

- **BUN**: Increased in dehydration, RI, GI bleed
- **Creatinine**: Increased measured: Bactrim, Tagamet, meat in diet
- **GFR**: AKA creatinine clearance: nl > 80, adjust meds if < 60, dialyze if < 10
  - *Formula*: (lean kg)(140 - age)(0.85 if female)/(72)(stable creatinine); nl: > 80
- **Glucose**: Often rises during stress; random > 200 = diabetes
  - *Low*: "SAD LIFE" (**S**epsis, **A**ddison, **D**rug, **L**iver, **I**nsulin, **F**ast, **E**tOH); Top Three: drug, EtOH, sepsis

ANION GAP ACIDOSIS LABS

See Table 2.4 here

■ "MUD PILES" (**M**ethanol, **U**remia, **D**KA, **P**araldehyde, **I**NH, **I**ron, **L**actate, **E**thylene glycol, **E**thanol, **S**alicylate)

■ "MAD CHILD" (**M**etformin, **M**otrin, **A**PAP, **D**apsone, **C**O, **C**yanide, **H**ydrogen sulfide, **I**odine, **L**actate, **D**iamox)

■ "SICKO LAB": Add-on labs (**S**alicylate, **I**ron, **C**arbon monoxide, **K**etones, **O**sms, **L**actate, **A**PAP, **B**lood gas)

■ **3 Ts**: Toluene, Theophylline, Tylenol

■ **Ketones**: Lab measures acetoacetic acid, but not beta hydroxybutyrate, which is more prevalent
   ● *DDx*: DKA, starvation, alcoholic ketoacidosis, ethylene glycol

■ **Lactate**: High > 2.2–2.5. Critical > 4; half-life = 20 min. Mortality estimate = Lactate x 5
   ● *DDx*: A: shock, CO, ischemia; B: liver failure, CA, Sz, DM, F, burn, TPN, meds (Metformin, HIV). Spurious: Prolonged tourniquet time (best not to use), not placed on ice, old tube used

ABGs AND ACID-BASE

Compensate = Compensation: HB overestimated by 4%

■ **Aa Gradient**: Normal is 5–15; Aa = $(760-47)(FiO_2) - (1.25)(pCO_2) - pO_2$

■ **Venous Gas**: WNL: pH: 7.31–7.41, pCO_2: 39–49, pO_2: 30–50. If venous pCO_2 < 45 then arterial pCO_2 < 50

■ **Alkalosis**: More dangerous than acidic; can cause AMS, Sz, dysrhythmia, ↓Ca, ↓K; pH >7.6 = danger

■ **Ventilators**: Adjust to pH not pCO_2 (especially if baseline changes: pregnancy, COPD, etc.)

TABLE 2.4.   Acidotic Conditions

Acidosis, Metabolic		Acidosis, Respiratory
ABG:	Bicar of 15→ pH: 7.25; bicarb of 5→ pH: 7.10 Compensate: pCO2 = 1.5 (bic) + 8 = last two digit pH	ABG: Acute = <36h: pCO2 of 50→pH of 7.32 　　　　　　　　pCO2 of 60→pH of 7.24 　　　　　　　　pCO2 of 70→pH of 7.16 　　　　　　　　pCO2 of 80→pH of 7.08 Chronic => 36hr: pCO2 of 50→pH of 7.37 　　　　　　　　pCO2 of 60→pH of 7.34 　　　　　　　　pCO2 of 70→pH of 7.31 　　　　　　　　pCO2 of 80→pH of 7.28
DDx:	Nongap: G.I. Nongap: Renal Diarrhea　　RTA, NH3, Diamox Fistula　　　Hypocapnia Neo-Bladder Anion Gap Acidosis: (Gap > 16) "MUD PILES" (Methanol, Uremia, DKA, Paraldehyde, INH, Iron, Lactate, Ethylene glycol, Ethanol, Salicylate) "MAD CHILD" (Metformin, Motrin, APAP, Dapsone, CO, Cyanide, Hydrogen sulfide, Iodine, Lactate, Diamox) "3Ts" (Toluene, Theophylline, Tylenol)	DDx: "SLOW" Sedation Lung problems COPD: Mostly pH 7.36–7.38 at baseline Weakness
Rx:	1° cause. Start vent č AC at two-thirds baseline RR	Rx: Albuterol, BiPAP, intubate, suction, etc.

TABLE 2.5.   Alkalotic Conditions

Alkalosis, Metabolic		Alkalosis, Respiratory	
ABG:	Bicarb of 25→ pH: 7.40 Bicarb of 35→ pH: 7.55 Compensate: bic↑10→ pCO2 ↑ 7, (max = 55)	ABG: Acute = < 36 hr: pCO2 of 30→ pH: 7.48 　　　　　　　　pCO2 of 20→ pH: 7.56 Chronic => 36 hr: pCO2 of 30→ pH: 7.43 　　　　　　　　pCO2 of 20→ pH: 7.46	
DDx:	Urine chloride < 10　　Urine chloride > 10 diuretic, diarrhea　　Conn's syndrome cystic fibrosis　　　Cushing's, steroid post-hypercapnia　　Barter's syndrome NG suction, vomiting　Hypokalemia	DDx: CNS　　　　　　　Pulmonary Anxiety, pain, ↑thyroid　PE CVA, pregnancy　　　CHF ASA　　　　　　　Pneumonia Fever, sepsis, shock　Hypoxia	
Rx:	GI: H2 blocker, NaCl > KCl > HCl > diamox GU: depends on cause: NS, K, Mg	Rx: Treat primary cause, benzodiazepines	

MIXED ACID-BASE DISORDER DECODING AND THE ΔΔ (DELTA-DELTA)

■ **1. Check pH and pCO_2**
  - *pH < 7.4 and pCO_2 > 40 = respiratory acidosis*
  - *pH > 7.4 and pCO_2 < 40 = respiratory alkalosis*
  - *pH > 7.4 and pCO_2 > 40 = metabolic alkalosis with respiratory compensation*
  - *pH < 7.4 and pCO_2 < 40 = metabolic acidosis with respiratory compensation*

■ **2. Check ΔΔ = Delta Gap**: This will tell you if there is a SECOND metabolic derangement.
  - *Calculate the Anion Gap (AG)*: $AG = Na - Cl - HCO_3$
  - *Subtract 10 (the average normal gap). This is the Base Excess*: $BE = AG - 10$
  - *Calculate the Delta Gap*: $ΔΔ = BE + HCO_3$
    - If ΔΔ ($BE + HCO_3$) is > 24 then there is an additional metabolic alkalosis
    - If ΔΔ ($BE + HCO_3$) is < 24 then there is an additional metabolic acidosis

Normal Values (Note: will vary lab to lab)	
Albumin	3.3–5.0
Alk phos	< 130
ALT	10–45
Ammonia	11–35
Amylase	30–150
Anion gap	8–15
AST	10–45
Bilirubin	< 1.2
BUN	8–18
Calcium	9.0–10.6
Chloride	97–107
Glucose	65–110
Ionized	1.13–1.32
LDH	< 175
Lipase	6–60
Magnesium	1.8–2.5
Osmolality	280–310
Phosphorus	2.5–4.5
Potassium	3.5–5.0
Sodium	135–145

Hemoglobin A1c	Average Glucose
5	100
6	125
7	150
8	185
9	210
10	240
11	270
12	300

LIVER FUNCTION TESTS

- **Albumin**: Half-life is 2–3 weeks, so can be a late finding
- **Alk Phos**: "BILP" (**B**one, **I**ntestine, **L**ung, **L**iver [GGT also up], **P**lacenta)
  - *Drugs*: Bactrim, Augmentin
  - *AP/ALT*: < 2: hepatitis. > 5: biliary obstruction, ameba
- **ALT**: "L = liver" (more specific for liver disease)
  - *DDx*: "HKLMN" (**H**eart, **K**idney, **L**iver, **M**uscle, **N**SAID)
  - *ALT > 1000*: Tox, virus, shock, rhabdomyolysis
- **AST**: "S = Stolichnaya vodka" and systemic (less specific for nonalcoholic liver disease)
  - *DDx*: HKLMN; NSAID; also pancreas, lung, WBCs, RBC
  - *AST > ALT*: Alcohol ("A Scotch and tonic"); if so, ratio usually about 2:1; rhabdomyolysis: CK = about 20 times the AST
- **Ammonia**: Can be normal in hepatic encephalopathy; can have delayed rise
  - *DDx*: Urea cycle defect, organic acidemia, liver failure, depakote, ASA, 5FU, asparaginase, TPN, Reye's syndrome, UTI from urease producing organism (proteus)
- **Bilirubin**: Direct < 15%: hemolysis, CHF, Gilbert's(bili 1.2–3-(5)), ppt: fasting, surgery, ID,EtOH, exertion. Direct > 30%: ID (u viral), tox, EtOH(AST/ALT > 1.5), obstructing mass
- **Pro Time**: No measurable change in PT until factor levels drop <50% baseline

PANCREAS PLUS

- **Amylase**: 85% sensitive, 70% specific. May be Nl in pancreatitis from EtOH/medication, ↑TG, sx >1wk. Can have ↑lipase with amylase < 50 or fatal pancreatitis with normal amylase.
  - *Kinetics*: Rise: 6–24h, Peak: 48h, Normalizes: 6d
  - *DDx*: Salivary = parotiditis, intestines, recurrent vomiting
- **Lipase**: 90% sensitive, 98% specific. More sensitive and specific than amylase
  - *Kinetics*: Rise: 4–8h, Peak: 24h, Normalizes: 11d
- **LDH**: RBC, lung (in PCP pneumonia usually > 300), liver, heart, muscle

ENDOCRINE

- **Cortisol**: Addison's, Cushing's; Normal: 2–20, but varies by time of day
- **Prolactin**: Sz, syncope > pseudo-seizure, sz meds
- **TSH**: WNL is 0.5–5, but if significant dz usually < 0.1 or > 10
- **T3 and T4**: Free T3 and T4 better to avoid errors due to altered thyroid binding globulin levels; can have pure T3 thyrotoxicosis
- **Beta HCG**: Urine + at 20 mIU/ml or 2 wks; false negative can occur if specific gravity < 1.015; serum + at 5–10 mIU/ml or 1-wk post-conception; false +: rheumatoid factor or certain antibodies, TOA, thyrotoxicosis, pituitary tumor; meds: aspirin, methadone, marijuana, antidepressants, antiepileptics; quant: 3–4 wk: 5–130, 4–5 wk: 75–2600, 5–6 wk: 850–20,000, 6–7 wk: 4000–100,000; doubling: weeks 2–5 doubles q1.5d; weeks 5–12: doubles q2–3d

CK, CARDIAC, AND VASCULAR LABS

- **Brain Natiuritic Peptide (BNP):** Rises with ventricular dilation; half-life = 30 min
  - *DDx:* CHF (FN: 1st hr, acute MR/MS), PE, CRF: Cr > 2.5, ACS, ESLD, PHTN, HRT, age, HTN with LVH, DM, hyperthyroid, Cushing's cirrhosis, SAH, paraneoplastic syndromes
  - *False pos.:* Tend to be higher in older women (esp. age > 75), higher in renal failure (cleared by kidney)
  - *False neg.:* First 1–2 hours (t½: 2 hr), obesity lowers level
  - *Levels:* < 100: "Normal," but 50–500 or 222–333 = gray zone: CHF uncertain, consider other Dx); 100–400: PE, cor pulmonale, class 1 CHF (if < 200 consider outpt; Rx), LVH, cirrhosis; > 400: acute CHF exacerbation or chronic class 2 CHF; > 600: predicts ↑mortality: > 600 = class 3 CHF; > 800 = class 4 CHF
- **Cholesterol:** LDL: CAD: < 100, DM or 2 RF: < 130, 1RF: < 160; if no RF and > 160:diet, > 190: drug
- **CK, Total:** Muscular dystrophy, seizure, myositis, rhabdo, drunk, electrocution, EMG, IM injection, surgery, AMI, EtOH, malignant hyperthermia, medication (statins, doxycycline)
  - *CK-MB:* Rise: 4–6 hr, peak 12–24 hr, duration 12–48 hr
  - *CK-index = CK-MB/CK-total:* > 5: suggests MI; 3–5: gray zone; < 3: unlikely MI
- **D-Dimer:** Whole blood: 85%/68%; ELISA: 97%/20%, takes 4 hr; latex: 70%/76%; immunoassay: 97%+; turbidimetric: > 95%, 2 hr point of care: 85–96%
  - > 250 ng/ml: Trauma: post-op 10d, bruise, peripartum/PIH; clot: DVT, PE, MI, CVA, dissection, AAA; chronic Dz: liver, renal, CA, DM, CVD, sickler; ID/inflammation: pericarditis, ID, DIC
  - < 250 ng/ml: False negatives: Sx > 1 wk, on heparin, on warfarin (of positives only 15–40% have PE/DVT)
- **Myoglobin:** Rise early, nonspecific; if doesn't double in 1–2 hr: 98% sensitive for MI, not ACS
- **Troponin I:** < 0.01 normal, unstable angina; 0.01–0.1 = gray zone (risk even if ESRD); > 0.1 = MI
  - *Timing:* Rise: 3–6 hr; peak: 18–24 hr; NI: 3–10d; hour/sensitivity: 0 hr/50%, 4 hr/75%, 8 hr/85%, 12 hr/99%, 18 hr/100%
  - *DDx:* Trauma, PTCA, OR, defib, carditis, low BP, PE, amyloid, thyroid dz, transplant rejection, dissection, heterophile Ab (constant: no rise and fall), vasospasm, sepsis, chemo, CVA, SAH
  - *C&T:* Troponin-C is nonspecific; Troponin-T can be elevated in renal failure; Troponin-I is best
- **Future?** Myeloperoxidase > 198pM for vulnerable plaques, ischemic-modified albumin: 75% for angina

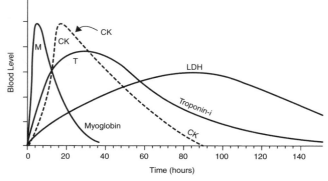

FIGURE 2.33. Hours from onset of myocardial infarction.

ANEMIA

Type and cross indications: shock, Hb < 10, to OR, active bleeding; o/w type and screen

■ **Normal Hemoglobin (Hb)**: Age 1 mon: 10–14; age 2 yr: 11–14; adults: male: 14–17, female: 12–16

■ **Hemoglobin Changes**: 1 unit PRBC > ↑ Hb by 1; dilution by 30 cc/kg > drop of Hb by 2 max

■ **Anemia**: Acute: ↑HR, nl MCV and RDW, ↑BUN; chronic: nl HR, low MCV, ↑RDW

■ **Retics**: Reticulocyte count x Hct/30 > 2?

■ **Hemolytic**: ↑LDH, ↑bili, ↑reticulocytes, ↑urobilinogen; hemoglobinuria, schistocytes, ↓haptoglobin. +Coombs: Coombs: indirect = Ab screen; direct = "DAT" (direct antibody test)
   ● *DDx*: Spherocytosis, HbS, Ab, med, tox, malaria, C. perf, TTP, HUS, DIC, PNH, G6PD, low Phos

■ **Macrocytic**: ↓Folate: EtOH, vegan, liver dz; ↓B$_{12}$: omeprazole, fish tapeworm, pernicious anemia, bowel resection; other: HIV meds

■ **Microcytic**: ↑ TIBC: ↓iron: anisocytosis, poikilocytosis, low Fe; NI TIBC: thalassemia (microcytosis out of proportion), sideroblastic anemia; low TIBC: chronic disease (most common in elderly: ↑ferritin, NI RDW)

■ **Normocytic**: Renal dz, chronic dz, acute bleed, hemolysis (see earlier Hemolytic section), other

TRANSFUSIONS: GET CONSENT!

■ **Indications**: Significant symptoms; CAD and Hb < 10; elderly and Hb < 9; acute bleed and Hb < 8; chronic and Hb < 7

■ **Precautions**: Wash: no IgA, neonate, PNH; leukocyte poor: transplant patient, prior reaction; radiated: ↓immune pt (can get grafts vs. host disease)

■ **Reactions**: Febrile > allergic > hemolytic > septic. Death: 1 in 100k. Reaction to O-neg: 1 in 150
   ● *Death*: Risk: 1 in 300,000 components = 1/45,000 recipients; TRALI > sepsis > hemolysis
   ● *Fever*: If fever stop blood, if r/o hemolysis (spin crit, haptoglobin, free Hb, CBC, Coombs) can continue

■ **Infections**: Table 2.6 shows risk per unit transfused: Bacteria > Chaga's > Parvovirus > Hepatitis B...
   ● *Others*: HTLV: 1 in 640,000; CMV, EBV, HDV, HGV, malaria, syphilis

TABLE 2.6. Risk for Various Diseases Per Unit of Blood Transfused

Disease	HIV	Hep A	Hep B	Hep C	ParvoB19	Bacteria	Babesia	Chaga's
Risk/unit	1:2 million	1:1 million	1:200,000	1:2 million	1:20,000	1:12,000	1:1 million	1:42,000

■ **Other Risks**: Hypothermia, volume overload

C-REACTIVE PROTEIN AND ERYTHROCYTE SEDIMENTATION RATE

■ **C-Reactive Protein (CRP)**: Rises earlier than ESR
   ● *Normal*: < 1.0. High: > 3.0; like ESR, nonspecific, but sensitive and good for measuring response to treatment

■ **Erythrocyte Sedimentation Rate (ESR)**: Less sensitive than CRP as rises more slowly
   ● *Normal*: Male WNL: 0–17 or < age/2; female WNL: 1–25 or < (age + 10)/2
   ● *DDx of ↑*: CVD, ID, inflam., malignancy, MI, thyroid, rouleaux, osteomyelitis, temporal arteritis, gout

WHITE BLOOD CELLS

- **Normal:** 4 –10 (or 11)
  - *Pediatric:* 1d–1 wk: 5–30; 1 wk–1 mon: 5–20, 60% lymphs; 1 mon–2 yr: 6–17.5; 2 yr–6 yr: 5–15; 6 yr–12 yr: 4.5–13.5; > 12 yr: 4–10
- **WBC Low**
  - *Infection:* CMV, viral, bacterial sepsis, HIV (CD4 = 20% lymphocyte count)
  - *Drug:* Gold, Tagamet, Indocin, PCN, phenothiazine, PTU, sulfa, Dilantin, ACEI, Zyvox
- **WBC High**
  - *Disease:* Infection, inflammation, cancer
  - *Other:* Stress, seizure, pain
  - *Drugs:* Cocaine, steroid
  - *Note:* Demargination can raise WBC up to 17,500 and band count up to 10%
- **Bandemia:** Normal varies by lab: < 5–11; bands >10 c/w sepsis
  - *DDx:* Sickle cell crisis, Sz, ID, pregnancy, GI bleed, chemo, Neupogen, Neumega
- **Metamyelocytes:** ID, CML, pernicious anemia, spleen, myelodisplasia, Neupogen, Neumega
- **Toxic Granulation:** Severe infection/inflammation: more specific and ominous but less sensitive than bands
- **Dohle Body:** Severe infection or inflammation: more ominous and more specific but less sensitive than bands
- **Leukemia:** Lymphoblast, myeloblast, promyelocyte, Auer rod = AML, smudge cells = CML or CLL
- **Atypical Lymphocytes:** EBV, CMV, toxoplasmosis, HIV, Hepatitis A&B, measles, mumps, rubella, roseola, drug rxn
- **Eosinophils**
  1. Infection: Cocci, HIV, worms (in immigrant assume worms: get O&P but treat empirically)
  2. Immune: Allergy/meds, Addison's, CVD, Crohn's, asthma, Churg-Strauss, Loffler's
  3. Cancer: Lymphoma, Ovarian, Hodgkin's
  4. Drugs: Sz meds, Sulfa, H2, INH
- **Monocytes:** TB, brucellosis, chronic inflammation
- **Basophils:** Parasite, CA, sarcoid

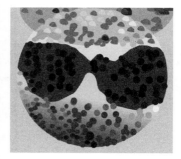

FIGURE 2.34.   Toxic granulation. Badness: Beware!

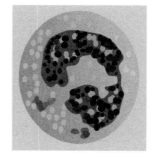

FIGURE 2.35.   Dohle bodies. Badness: Beware!

PLATELETS

- ■ **Platelets High**: Inflam, ID, visceral CA, bleed, low Fe, CA, PCV, CML, ET (essential thrombocythemia); reactive (GIB, ID, pancreatitis, cirrhosis), post-splenectomy, ↓iron, postpartum; CA (PCV, CML, GI, myelofibrosis, essential thrombocytosis)
- ■ **Platelets Low**: DIC, HUS, artifact, drugs, ITP, TTP, pancytopenia, etc.
  - *Transfuse*: Platelets < 10–20K: Give prophylactically unless ITP or TTP; platelets < 50K: Give if actively bleeding. Consider if ESLD, p chemo, ↑INR, ESRD

COAGULATION TESTS

Coagulation	WNL	Notes/Therapeutic Levels
Platelet function test	Has replaced the bleeding time	90% sensitive for vWD
Factors	60–140%	Low in hemophilia, liver disease, warfarin
Ristocetin cofactor	75–125%	Most sensitive test for Von Willebrand's disease (except type IID)
PT and PTT both ↑		DDx: Leptirudin, agatroban, all those following, error (short tube, delay, etc.)
Pro time	11–13 sec	DDx: Liver dz, vit K deficiency, factor deficit or inhibitor, warfarin, DIC
		Rx: INR goals: 2.0–3.0: for most conditions: PE, DVT, A-fib, etc.; 2.5–3.5: for metal valve, APLS
		INR > 5 is risky; INR > 20 admit (if 7:1 in 100 risk comp in 48 hr)
PTT	22–35 sec	DDx: Lupus anticoagulant, factor deficiency or inhibitor, heparin; factors: 12, 11, 8 (hemophilia A), 9 (hemophilia B), von Willebrand's

TABLE 2.7　PTT Goals for Heparin Therapy

Disease	PTT Goal	Measured PTT	Infusion Hold	Rate Δ	Repeat PTT
PE/DVT	**59–88**	< 48	none	↑3.5 u/k/h	4 hr
		48–58	none	↑1.5 u/k/h	4 hr
		89–101	60 min	↓1.5 u/k/h	4 hr
		> 101	60 min	↓3.5 u/k/h	4 hr
ACS	**52–76**	< 38	none	↑4 u/k/h	4 hr
		38–51	none	↑2 u/k/h	4 hr
		77–94	none	↓2 u/k/h	4 hr
		> 94	60 min	↓3 u/k/h	4 hr
NOTE: PTT goals may vary. Some newer guidelines recommend goal of 78–115 sec for DVT/A-fib and 70–101 sec for ACS or high risk for bleeding.					

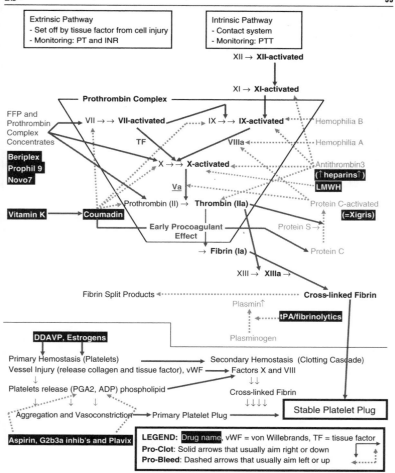

FIGURE 2.36. Coagulation and hemostatis.

GENERAL TOXICOLOGY TESTING

■ **Anion Gap**
- "MUDPILETS" (**M**ethanol, **P**araldehyde, **I**ron, **INH**, **E**tOH, **T**oluene [glue], **S**alicylate)
- "MAD CHILD" (**M**etformin, **A**PAP, **D**apsone, **C**O/CN, **C**olchicine, **H**. sulfide, **I**odine, **D**iamox)

■ **Drug Levels**: Assume patient is laying: get a 2nd level 3 hours later to document dropping

■ **EKG**
- *Long QT*: Cocaine, phenothiazines, TCAs, amiodarone, arsenic, cisapride, biaxin, EES, pentamidine, tacrolimus, methadone, astemizole, cardiac meds
- *RBBB*: TCAs, anticholinergics, propoxyphene, sodium channel blockers

■ **Osmolality Gap**: Methanol and ethylene glycol have pure osm gap early, then mixed, and finally only an anion gap

■ **Urine Tox**: Rarely affects management or solves issues; 25% false positive and 25% false negative
- *False (-)*: Opiates: Methadone, Darvon, Percocet, Fentanyl; Benzos: Klonipin, Rohypnol, Ativan; Others: XTC, LSD, GHB, ketamine
- *False (+)*: Amphetamines: diet pills, cold meds; PCP: Dextromethorphan, flexeril, TCA; Opiates: Rifampin, levaquin, poppy seeds

SPECIFIC DRUGS AND TOXINS

■ **Acetaminophen**: May be asymptomatic so test
- *Normal*: Therapeutic: 5–20
- *Toxic*: Hour post-OD and serum level to initiate NAC for acute ingestion; Note: May be toxic even if level < line: ↑LFTs (u > 8 hr), dose > 150 mg/k (10 g), half-life > 3 hr, ↑p450, or malnourished
- *Time/Level*: Hour post-OD and serum level to initiate Rx for ACUTE ingestion (Therapeutic range is 5–20)

TABLE 2.8.   Minimum Tylenol Level Requiring Treatment After Acute Ingestion by Hours Post-Ingestion

Hours	4	5	6	7	8	9	10	11	12	13	14	15	16	18	20	24
Level (mcg/ml)	140	120	100	80	70	60	50	40	35	30	25	20	16	12	8	4

Source: Pregerson DB. *Quick Essentials Emergency Medicine 4.0.* ERPocketbooks.com; 2010:197.

■ **Dilantin**: Indications: Seizure, V-tach, digoxin toxicity
- *Normal*: Therapeutic: 10–20; zero order kinetics = small dose change > ↑↑level
- *Correction*: Dilantin is 90% protein bound; effective level = measured level/(0.9)(serum albumin/4.4)
- *Levels*: 20: Nystagmus; 30: Ataxia, slurred speech, N/V; 40: AMS. 90: Coma, Sz, cardiac tox rare
- *Dispo*: Admit: Level > 25, increasing level, ataxia

■ **Digoxin**: Indications: CHF + A-fib
- *Normal*: Therapeutic: 0.5–2.2 (0.7–0.9 thought to be ideal)
- *Dispo*: ICU: OD and level > 2; digibind indicated for level > 10; Tele: Chronic level > 2.5

■ **Lithium**: Indications: Bipolar disorder
- *Normal*: Therapeutic: 0.5–1.5
- *Toxic*: Dialyze: Level > 4 acute; > 2.5 chronic; > 1.5 + moderate sx, ESRD

■ **Theophylline**: Indications: End-stage COPD refractory to other therapies
- *Normal*: Therapeutic: 10–20; Levels ↑by: Cipro, EES, H2 blockers, flu shot
- *Toxic*: Dialyze: Level > 100 acute or > 60 chronic
- *Dispo*: Admit: Level > 100 acute, > 30 or rising level; Home: If level < 30 and dropping consider home

■ **Valproate**: Indications: Seizure, bipolar disorder, migraine headaches
- *Normal*: Therapeutic: 50–100
- *Toxic*: Level > 150 get labs (LFTs, amylase)

URINE DIP

- ■ **General**: Wait for the micro; dip alone may lead you astray—but then so may the micro
- ■ **Normal**: Sg: 1.001–1.035, pH: 5–8, trace urobilinogen
- ■ **Beta HCG**: Should be neg > 2wk s/p abortion; sensitivity is 99.4% (but if dilute urine use 20 drops)
- ■ **Glucose**: Serum glucose > 180, Fanconi syndrome, multiple myeloma
- ■ **Heme**: False +: pH > 9, semen, myoglobin
- ■ **Leukocyte Esterase (LE)**: 85%/80% for UTI
- ■ **Nitrites**: 50/98 for UTI (if positive usually E. coli or Klebsiella)
- ■ **Protein**: Prot: 1+ = 30; 2+ = 100; 3+ = 300; 4+ = 2000; 3+ is bad.; IV contrast causes false elevation
  - ● *DDx*: DM, Glomerular dz; if hematuria too worry: vasculitis > rapid ARF
- ■ **Reducing Substances**: Galactosemia, amino-acidopathy, organic acidemia
- ■ **Sodium**: <10: Dehydration, low Na, prerenal; >20: SIADH, ATN

URINE MICRO

- ■ **Normal**: < 3 RBC, < 5 WBC, < 5 epi's (< 10 ok for woman), occ. hyaline or epithel casts
- ■ **Colors**
  - ● *Dark/Brown*: Porphyria, melanoma, rhabdomyolysis, bile, cascara, iron, macrobid
  - ● *Red*: Blood, beets, food coloring, myoglobin, urate, blackberries, dyes, serratia, fava; meds: cascara, doxorubicin, chloroquine, deferoxamin, ibuprofen, iron, macrobid
  - ● *Orange*: Pyridium, rifampin, bile, carrots, rhubarb, sulfa, fluoresceine, vitamin A/B_{12}
  - ● *Green/Blue*: Biliverdin, methylene blue, food color, pseudomonas, Elavil, Robaxin, Tagamet; blue diaper syndrome (tryptophan), triamterene, Doan's kidney pills
  - ● *Purple*: Alkali urine with klebsiella or pseudomonas UTI
- ■ **RBCs**: Worry if ↑Cr or protein; kidney stone, glomerular dz (dysmorphic), Normal, CA, ID, PCKD
  - ● *DDx*: Age < 20 yr: AGN, UTI, congenital, HUS. 20–60: UTI > CA > stone > PCKD. > 60: UTI > BPH > CA
  - ● *Benign*: After exercise (common), sex, menses, mild trauma
- ■ **WBCs**: 75–96% sensitive and 70–80% specific for UTI. If RBC > WBC in UTI, consider kidney stone
  - ● *DDx*: UTI, STD, GU-TB, AIN, SLE, IUP, prostatitis, kidney stone, nephritis, discitis/osteomyelitis; psoas abscess, diverticulitis, papillary necrosis, appy, tic, fistula, lymphoma
- ■ **Bacteria**: 55% sensitive and 90% specific for UTI
  - ● *DDx*: Contamination, UTI (even if no pyuria)
  - ● *Asx*: Rate about 5%. Rx if pregnant, pre-op GU, granulocytopenia or renal transplant, but not DM
- ■ **Other Cells**
  - ● *Epithelial*: Contamination (> 5/hpf for man, > 10/hpf for woman) >> ATN, papillitis, nephritis
  - ● *Transitional*: Large numbers may be from malignancy
  - ● *WBC/Glitter*: ID, GU-TB, tumor, GN, XRT, interstitial nephritis, chlamydia
- ■ **Casts**
  - ● *Hyaline*: Devoid of cells: < 5–10/hpf is WNL
  - ● *Granular*: ATN
  - ● *Hyaline*: HTN, nephrotic, dehydration, exercise
  - ● *Waxy*: CRF, amyloid
  - ● *Broad*: CRF
  - ● *Fatty*: Nephrotic, DM
  - ● *RBC Casts*: Nephritis, SLE, SBE, malignant HTN
  - ● *WBC Casts*: Pyelo, nephritis
- ■ **Crystals**
  - ● *Benign*: Amorphous, calcium oxalate and uric acid all usually benign
  - ● *Bad*: Cysteine, leusine, tyrosine

URINE CULTURE

- ■ **Contaminant**: Mixed flora, lactobacillus, alpha hemolytic strep, diptheroids, coag(-)staph
- ■ **Pathogenic**: Single strain, usually > 10,000–100,000 colonies/ml

STOOL GUAIAC CARD

- *How to*: Wait 3 minutes before adding developer. Add to specimen box first.
- *False positive*: Red meat, iron (50%), turnips, artichoke, broccoli, banana, grapes
- *Black stool and neg.*: Pepto-Bismol, iron (50%), charcoal, licorice
- *False negative*: Slow bleed (miss > 33% CA), high-dose vitamin C, antacids; stomach acid (use a gastro-cult card instead)

STOOL: INFECTION

- *Fecal WBC*: 73/84 for invasive diarrhea
- *C. dif. toxin*: Low sensitivity: Do at least three times before considering negative.
- *Lactoferrin*: 92/79 for invasive diarrhea
- *Rotavirus*: Stool DFA

STOOL CULTURE

- *Normal flora*: Enterobacteiaceae, strep, pseudomonas, yeast, staph
- *Pathogenic*: Salmonella, shigella, campylobacter, E. coli 0157:H7, yersinia
- *Special media*: Yersinia, vibrio, E. coli 0157:H7

STOOL: OTHER

- *DNA panel*: Four times more sensitive than guaiac for colon cancer
- *Apt test*: Tells fetal vs. maternal blood. Can use in GI bleed w/u to see if from cracked nipples.

BLOOD CULTURES

- *Technique*: Alcohol swipe lid, don't change needle, do 2–3 BCx (different site, same time OK); need minimum of 10 ml blood (but 42 ml of blood in one bottle better than two cultures)
- *Don't do*: If already gave ABX in the ED (if on orals at home yes on BCx)
- *True (+)*: About 10% of all blood cultures are true positives and 10% of those change management
- *False (+)*: Usually: Diptheroids (gram+ rods), coag neg. staph (epidermidis, warneri), gamma-strep. Often: Corynebacterium, proproprionibacterium, bacillus, viridans strep. Rates: 1+/2 bottles: 80% false positive; 1+/1 bottle: 45% false (+); 2+/2 (dif sites): 3% false (+); current contamination rates are lower: usually ~3% in ED and ~1.5% hospital wide

OTHER CULTURES

To avoid skin contamination wipe away excess pus first

- ■ **Ear Culture**: Wipe then aim swab for TM and avoid touching sides
- ■ **Eye Culture**: Wipe then swab inside lower lid
  - *Cornea*: Technique: Dip cotton swab in thio-broth, swab ulcer, plate (blood and chocolate agar), Q-tip in broth
- ■ **Throat Culture**: Technique: Swab purulent area if worried about GC, need to use Thayer-Martin media
- ■ **Viral**: Technique: Nasal washing in infants; nasal (throat) swab in others. Takes 3–10 days
- ■ **Wound Culture**: Technique: Wipe, clean with betadine, express fresh pus, then swab.

TABLE 2.9.   Culture Results

Shape	Gram Stain	Possible Pathogenic Strains and Diseases
Cocci	Gram-negative	Neisseria, Moraxella
	Gram-positive chains and pairs	β-hemolytic Strep Group A: pyogenes: strep throat, cellulitis, necrotizing fasciitis Group B: agalactiea: vaginal flora: neonate sepsis, CNS Group D: fecalis = enterococcus, bovis (is alpha or nonhemolytic) α-hemolytic Strep Pneumococcus: lung, bacteremia, CNS, ENT Viridans(mitis and mutans): endocarditis, bovis (a group D strep)
	Gram positive in clusters	Staph aureus: coagulase positive Staph epidermidis: coagulase negative (usually a contaminant)
Coccobacilli	Gram-negative?	Haemophilus influenzae, Haiemophilus ducreyi
Bacilli	Gram-positive	Corynebacteria, Listeria, Bacillus, Clostridia, Actinomyces, Nocardia
	Gram-negative	**GI:** E. coli, Salmonella, Shigella, Vibrio, Campylobacter. **Lung:** Klebsiella, Enterobacter, Serratia, Pseudomonas, Morganella, Hemophilus, Legionella, Bordetella **Zoonoses:** Brucella, Pasteurella, Yersinia
Anaerobes	N/A	Actinomyces, Bacteroides, Clostridia, Fusobacteria,Peptostretococci
No cell wall	N/A	Chlamydia, Coxiella, Mycoplasma, Rickettsia, Ureaplasma
Spirochetes	N/A	Borrelia, Treponema

IMMUNOLOGIC TESTS

■ **Cold Agglutinin:** Mycoplasma: 80% +: put 0.3 cc blood in a blue top, then on ice x 30 sec; cryoglobulinemia causes: Hep C, RA, SLE, leukemia, mycoplasma

■ **Direct Fluorescent Antibody (DFA):** Fluorescent molecule linked to antibody added then washed. Add DFA agent; wash. If antigen tested for is present, can see fluorescence by microscope. Results take hours. Some are: influenza A and B, parainfluenza, RSV, adenovirus

■ **Enzyme-Linked Immunosorbent-Assay (EIA/ELISA):** Ab linked to enzyme that changes color of reagent. It doesn't wash away if antigen tested for is present and so there is a positive color change. Automated with spectrophotometer = 1 hr-turnaround: RSV, influenza

■ **Malaria:** Binax NOW: Detects falciparum (most fatal): 95% and vivax (#1 cause): 87%.

■ **Polymerase Chain Reaction (PCR):** Cell lysed for DNA, which is then hugely amplified and detected.

■ **Peptide Nucleic Acid Fluorescence in Situ Hybridization (PNA FISH):** IDs organism w/in hours of +Cx; staph aureus: G+ cocci in clusters: positive = S. aureus. negative = other; enterococcus: G+ cocci in pairs and chains: positive = enterococci. negative = other; Candida: yeast: positive = C. albicans (use fluconazole). negative = other (use other meds)

■ **PPD:** Read at 48–72 hr. Only measure induration. 5 mm: HIV, recent contacts with TB, ↓immunity. 10 mm: IVDU, high-risk setting (travel, work), age < 4 yr. 15 mm: No known risks for TB.
  ● *False:* FN = 15%: recent infection (3–12 wk delay), anergy, miliary TB. FP: BCG, related mycobacteria

■ **Quantiferon:** Alternate to PPD. Quantitative. May eventually replace the PPD

■ **Serology:** Tests serum for concentration of antibody against a disease organism; positive test usually requires a four-fold rise in antibody titer

STD TESTING

■ **Men**: Urine amplified GC and chlamydia probe OK; should be done on initial stream urine

■ **Women**: Cervical specimens more sensitive. If urine, must be on unwiped initial stream

■ **Chlamydia**

- *Culture*: 50–90%/99%, expensive
- *DFA*: 80%/99%, expensive
- *POC*: 83%/99%
- *PCR*: 92–95% (but 80–85% on urine in women)/99%
- *EIA*: 40–60%/99%

■ **Herpes**: Viral Cx (not Ab): 95% if blister. Tzanck not great. IgG: + in prior infection

■ **Syphilis**: Dark-field microscopy, serologic tests

- *RPR/VDRL*: Serum nontreponemal tests; quantitative so can follow for cure (a four-fold drop in titer); less specific: false neg: early dz (do dark-field and repeat in 2 wk), late dz (do FTA-ABS); less sensitive: false pos: autoimmune dz
- *FTA-ABS*: Serum treponemal test. Qualitative, so cannot track level and it stays positive after cure; more specific and more sensitive than RPR/VDRL, but not as specific for active disease

SKIN MICROSCOPY

■ **Scabies**

- Find burrow; put two drops of ink on it to seep into burrow, then wipe with alcohol pad.
- Add a drop of mineral oil under nails, then scrape with 15 blade until flecks of blood appear.
- Place specimen on slide with cover slip and examine at 10x magnification for mites and eggs.

■ **KOH**: Must gently heat over Bunsen two to three passes. On the skin, a single hypha is diagnostic

■ **Tzanck**: Unroof vesicle, scrape floor, smear on slide, air dry, fix, stain, rinse. +: giant cell c̄8–10 nuclei

■ **Woods Lamp**: Red: Cornybacterium; Green: Tinea microsporum; Orange: Tinea versicolor

RADIATION RISKS

■ General Consideration

- *Exposure*: Increasing each year due to increased imaging, 30% of which is likely unnecessary
- *Risks*: Cancer, intellect. Dose/risk is cumulative over lifetime. No minimum safe dose. Studies: BEIR VII. Cancer: Information is extrapolated/estimated from higher dose exposures, so actual risk unknown. Top types: Leukemia: 2–5 yr latency; thyroid and breast: 10–20 yr latency
- *Benefits*: Usually outweigh risks, but as the threshold for CT scans drops, this may not always be true
- *Dose*: Varies significantly based on study, machine, manufacturer, body habitus, technique, etc.
- *Background*: 2.4–3.6 mSv/year from cosmic rays, terrestrial gamma rays, inhalation of radon, etc.
- *Body part*: Risks of cancer higher for head, neck, and torso; less for CXR and extremities
- *Age*: After age 60, risk is very small. Children at 10 times higher risk because rapidly dividing cells and longer life expectancy.

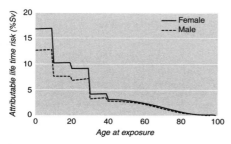

FIGURE 2.37.   Graph of how radiation risk decreases with age.
Courtesy of Eugenio Picano, MD.

- *Pregnancy*: Minimize exposure. However, ACOG states up to 50 mSv cumulative dose is acceptable. This is the dose TO THE FETUS, which varies depending on month of gestation. Equivalent dose to fetus is significantly more than dose to the mother.
- *Necessity*: 30% of diagnostic imaging thought to be unnecessary. Worry less well age > 65
  IN THE NEWS: In the US, it is estimated that the radiation exposure from the 62 million CT scans done annually may be responsible for 2% of all cancers in the future, researchers say in the *New England Journal of Medicine*. Because doctors underestimate the radiation risk from CT scans, they may be ordering too many of the scans. "If it is true that about one-third of all CT scans are not justified by medical need, and it appears to be likely, perhaps 20 million adults and, crucially, more than 1 million children per year in the United States are being irradiated unnecessarily."
- *No study*: Consider observation for nonspecific abdominal pain, head injury with brief LOC only; in classic appy cases, go to OR without CT.
- *Alternates*: Ultrasound and MRI have no known radiation. Use ultrasound first for peds RLQ pain; VQ or Ddimer preferred in young women with r/o PE. Peds dosing
- *Shielding*: Use lead shields for thyroid, fetus, gonads, etc., whenever possible.
- *Nuclear*: Thallium > Sestamibi > VQ scan. Tracer collects in bladder (near fetal head) so urinate often. For more info see: www.ccohs.ca/oshanswers/phys_agents/ionizing.html

■ RADIATION BASICS

- *Background*: Average dose = 3.6 mSv/year, 80% from nature (uranium, radium, radon, cosmic rays)
- *Nonionizing*: Radiation lacking energy to liberate orbital electrons (most of electromagnetic spectrum)
- *Ionizing*: High Energy: Has the ability to break chemical bonds, produce an ion pair, and damage DNA. Types: Particulate: Alpha particles, electrons = beta particles, neutrons, protons. Electromagnetic: X-rays, gamma rays (from nuclear medicine studies)

TABLE 2.10. The Electromagnetic Spectrum

EM Spectrum	Radio Waves	Microwave	Infrared Waves	Visible Spectrum	Ultraviolet	X-rays	Gamma Rays
Wavelength Size	Building, Human	Insect	Eye of a needle	Bacteria, Virus	Protein	Atom	Atomic nucleus
Frequency	Lowest	Lower	Low	Mid-range	High	Higher	Highest
Ionizing?	No	No	No	No	No	Yes	Yes

- **Units**: Biologic effects of different types of radiation vary; type and total absorbed dose matter. Gray (Gy): An absorbed dose measurement: Gray is expressed as J/kg. One gray is equal to 100 rad. Rad: Radiation absorbed dose. Also an absorbed dose measurement: For XR: 1 rad = 10 mSv. Sievert (Sv): Equivalent dose calculated by multiplying rads by a weight factor (i.e.: X-rays = 1, alpha = 20). Rem: Roentgen equivalents nan: an "equivalent dose": 1 rem = 10 milliSieverts. Others: Becquerels, Curies, amperes

- **Comparative Radiation Doses from Diagnostic Imaging**
  - *For XR*: 1 rad = 10mSv. Table 2.11 is helpful for comparison. Actual doses may vary (by more than ten-fold for CT). Doses in the literature for variety of tests vary significantly. Higher resolution (multidetector scanner, higher beam intensity, narrower slices) requires higher dosing.

TABLE 2.11. Comparative Radiation Doses from Diagnostic Imaging

Diagnostic Imaging Study	Average Dose (in milliSieverts)	Equivalent Dose (in CXRs)	Time for Equal Background Dose
Dental bite-wing	0.01	0.5	1d
Knee, ankle, elbow, wrist	0.02	1	2d
PA CXR	0.02	1	2d
Lateral CXR	0.04	2	4d
Skull	0.07	3.5	7d
C-spine series	0.3	15	1 mon
Mammogram	0.6	30	2 mon
KUB	0.6	30	2 mon
Pelvis/Hip	1.2	60	4 mon
CT (head)	2.0	100	8 mon
L-spine series	2.0	100	8 mon
V/Q scan	2.0	100	8 mon
IVP	3.0	150	1 yr
Yearly background exposure	3.0	150	1 yr
HIDA scan	3.7	185	1.2 yr
Bone scan	4.4	220	1.5 yr
PET scan	5–14	250–700	1.5–5 yr
Technetium sestamibi scan	6–12	300–600	2–4 yr
Cardiac cath +/- PTCA	5–50	250–2500	1.5–15 yr
CT (chest)	8–16	400–800+	2.5–5 yr
Barium enema	8	400	2.5 yr
Estimated dose causing 1 In 1000 risk of death	10	500	3 Yrs
CT (coronary)	10	500	3 yr
CT (abdomen and pelvis)	15–20	750–1000	5–7 yr
CT (urogram)	20	1000	7 yr
Thallium scan	12–24	600–1200	4–8 yr
IR procedures	25	1250	8 yr
Gallium scan	40	2000	13 yr

X-RAYS

■ **General**: Doses are cumulative with no minimum safe dose.

■ **Intellect**: Swedish army study for radiation of facial hemangiomas: the higher the dose of radiation, the lower the chance of attending high school. (Hall P, Adami HO, Trichopoulos D. Effect of low doses of ionising radiation in infancy on cognitive function in adulthood: Swedish population based cohort study. *BMJ*. 2004;328:19.)

■ **Cancer**: The most well-known delayed complication of radiation exposure is malignancy.

  • *Data*: Chernobyl, atomic bomb testing and survivors, medical radiation therapy, radium watch painters.

  • *Organs*: Can be any, but the worst are: thyroid CA, leukemia, breast cancer.

  • *Risk*: The lifetime risk of fatal cancer is estimated as follows in a *BMJ* study by Picano: > 1 in 2000: thallium > fluoroscopy > cardiac angiogram > Sestamibi > abdominal CT > 1 in 20,000: chest CT, barium enema, bone scan, lung scan

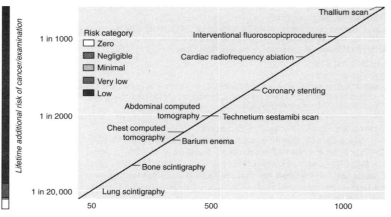

FIGURE 2.38. Radiation doses and cancer risk for various imaging tests.
Courtesy of Eugenio Picano, MD.

■ **Imaging in Pregnancy and ACOG Recommendations**

  • *Consider informed consent.*

  • *Note*: Effective doses to fetus are NOT the same as the effective dose to the mother, therefore, the following numbers DO NOT agree with Table 2.11

  • *Basics*: Risk mostly < 17 wks. Up to 5 rad is OK and probably up to 10–15 without malformation. Exposure is CUMULATIVE so ask about prior imaging. The 5 rad cumulative dose deemed acceptable by ACOG address risk for fetal abnormalities. The lifetime risk of cancer is not addressed by these guidelines, but the fetus is at high risk.

  • *Ultrasound*: Preferred imaging in pregnancy. Good for ectopic, pelvis, renal. Fair for appendicitis.

  • *MRI*: Good for appy, pelvic DVT, SBO, renal colic. Avoid gadolinium, especially in the 1st trimester.

  • *5 Rad Cutoff*: The following is the number of studies you would need to get to reach 5 rad = 50 mSv for fetus.
    Plain films: C-spine: 2500, chest: 70,000, LS-spine: 13, pelvis: 125, abdo: 13, BE:1, upper GI: 89, IVP: 3
    CT scan: head: 100, chest: 50 (Less rads to baby than VQ, but more to mom), abdo: 1, L-spine: 1
    VQ: VQ: 23. Perfusion only: 28. Do perfusion only. If +, then do ventilation.
    URINATE FREQUENTLY or Foley because tracer concentrates in the bladder (near the fetal head)

SKULL X-RAYS

- **Indications**: Rarely used as CT scanning much more sensitive for important findings. Some experts feel skull films in peds are more sensitive for certain fractures. Add to CT.
- **Fracture**: Sharp, straight, angles, asymmetric, nonsclerotic margins, nontapering, black not gray
- **Vessels**: Smooth, undulating, branching, sclerotic margins, tapering, gray not black
- **Findings**: Fractures, fluid level in sphenoid sinus, shifted midline structures, intracranial air

FACE X-RAYS

- **Indications**: Rarely used as CT scanning much more sensitive
- **Findings**: Asymmetry, abnormal "elephant's trunk" appearance of zygomatic arch, fluid in sinus
- **Mandible**: Ring-like so usually two fractures or fracture + dislocation; consider panorex view if available

NECK–SOFT TISSUE X-RAYS

- **Technique**: Inspiratory with neck extended and mouth closed. Be sure to do in extension while not crying or can get false positive soft tissue swelling.
- **Valecula Sign**: For epiglottitis: 98%/99%. Trace the base of the tongue to the hyoid bone; Valecula = air pocket between tongue base and epiglottitis; should be deep and near vertical.
- **Steeple Sign**: Narrowing of subglottic airway on AP view seen in croup

CERVICAL–SPINE X-RAYS

Only 2% positive for injury

- **NEXUS Tool**: Study had 818 fractures; of these there were eight misses and two were significant. (Mower WR, Hoffman JR, Herbert M. Developing a decision instrument to guide computed tomographic imaging of blunt head injury patients. *J Trauma.* 2005;59(4):954–959.)
  - *Criteria*: 1. No drugs/distracting injury, A + 0x4; 2. No neuro deficit; 3. Neck nontender midline
- **Canada Tool**: Exclusion: AMS, age < 16, OB, paralysis
  - *High risk*: Age > 65, parasthesias, mechanism (fall > 3ft, axial load, bad MVA, bike/ATV, rollover)
  - *Low risk*: Simple rear-end MVA or ambulatory or delayed pain or no midline tenderness
  - *Motion*: Able to rotate neck actively 45° L and R
- **Basics**: Lateral most important view. Make sure you see T1. X-rays may miss important injuries.
- **4-Lines**: Anterior and posterior spinal, spinolaminar, soft tissue (6 mm at C2, 22 mm at C6); lordotic or straight OK, but not kyphotic
- **Disk Space**: If wide, likely abnormal from hematoma, especially in elderly
- **Distances**: Dens to Chamberlain's line > 4 mm, > 11° angulation = ligamentous injury, > 2 mm subluxation; midmens to basion = 5 mm. Line down posterior clivus should barely touch odontoid
  - *Predental*: < 3 mm in adult, < 4.5 mm in child
  - *Pediatric*: Predental space up to 4.5 mm is OK. Pseudosubluxation < 2 mm may occur.
- **Flex-Ex**: In NEXUS, not very useful. Some say standard to r/o ligament injury. Must monitor patient.
- **Odontoid**: Lateral masses should line up
- **Unstable**: "Jefferson Bit Off a Hangman's Tit" (Jefferson, bilateral facet, burst, odontoid, any fx/dlc, hangman's, teardrop)
- **CT Scan**: More sensitive than plain films
- **Indications:** Coma, high suspicion (already getting a CT head), any fx seen on plain films

CHEST X-RAY

"ABCDs" (**A**irway, **B**ones/PTX, **C**ardiac/Mediastinum, **D**iaphragm, **S**oft Tissue)

- ■ **Indications**: Cough and fever with any of: age > 65 or < 4, RR > 24, HR > 100 in adult; abnormal pulse ox or auscultation; many others
- ■ **Adequate**: Right patient, exposure: should be able to see disc spaces and vessels behind heart; Inspiration: Six ribs anterior above diaphragm? Nine ribs posterior? "Nine is fine." Rotation
- ■ **False Neg.**: Immunosuppresion, PCP, TB, PE, dehydration
- ■ **Repeat**: Always repeat an abnormal CXR to check for resolution. If not, you could miss cancer.
- ■ **Pediatrics**: Anterior PTX: Medial lucency; heart size changes with volume status
- ■ **Airspace**: White: ATX, HTX, rotation, infiltrate, CHF, infarct. Dark-side: PTX, PE (oligemia), rotation
  - *ATX*: DDx: Splinting, CA, PNA, TB, fungi, inflammation, PE
  - *Cavitation*: Cancer, anaerobe, TB, staph, MRSA, Klebsiella
  - *CHF*: A: Alveolar infiltrates; B: Batwing infiltrates; C: CM, cuffing, cephalization
  - *PE*: Oligemia, lung volume, hemidiaphragm↑, ATX, infarct: effusion, infiltrate
  - *Reticular*: Fibrosis (lower and peripheral), sarcoid (esp. mid and upper reticulonodular)
  - *Nodules*: Small: TB, fungi, mycoplasma, measles. Medium: OGD (if no Ca++ must r/o CA). Multiple: CA, septic emboli, fungi > Wegeners, sarcoid, RA, AV fistula
- ■ **Bones**: Look for lytic lesions, Rib Fx, old Fx
  - *Trauma*: HTX: Decubitus more sensitive. PTX: Deep sulcus sign. Diaphragm rupture
- ■ **Cardiac/Mediastinum**

Esophagus, bronchi, nodes, nerves, aorta

  - *Curves*: Right Side: Bronchocephalic vessels, ascending aorta, right atrium, IVC. Left Side: Bronchocephalics, aortic arch, pulmonary art., left atrium, left ventricle.
  - *Masses*: 4 Ts: Teratoma, Thymoma, Thyroid goiter, Terrible lymphoma
  - *Nodes*: CA, sarcoid, lymphoma, TB, fungus, silicosis, pneumoconiosis
  - *Dissection*: Wide mediastinum, AP window, Ca++ in aorta displaced, ↑heart, left sided effusion, nl
  - *Boot heart*: LV aneurysm, effusion, tetrology of Fallot
- ■ **Diaphragm**

Normally should see both on AP and lateral views; R hemidiaphragm higher due to liver

  - *Free air*: CXR < 40% sensitive from free air in abdomen. Lateral is more sensitive.
  - *Effusion*: CA, CHF (R > L), PNA, TB, viral, ascites, pancreatitis, CVD, dissection, esophagus
  - *Elevation*: Phrenic nerve, lung, splinting, PE, pleura, trauma, scoliosis, HD rupture, organomegaly
  - *Injury*: Left PTX, basal opacity, loss of HD contour, shift of MS, elevated left hemidiaphragm
- ■ **Pulmonary Nodule**

Definition: < 3 cm, no LAN. Management may include: CT, observation (PET scan, Bx)

  - *DDx*: CA, OGD, benign, etc. Bad Px: change from old CXR, no Ca+
- ■ **TB**
  - *Miliary*: Diffuse 1–2 mm nodules with hilar adenopathy. DDx: fungi, viral, CA, atypical
  - *Primary*: Infiltrate, ATX, nodes, effusion, miliary (can appear normal)
  - *Reactivation*: Upper lobe, cavitary, nodular, pleural thickening, volume loss, bronchiectasis
- ■ **Procedures**
  - *ET tube*: Tip 5 cm above carina (chin in neutral)
  - *NG tube*: Tip in stomach
  - *Pacer lead*: Tip in apex of R ventricle
  - *Central line*: Tip in SVC

KUB/ABDOMINAL SERIES

- **Indications**: Concern for: obstruction (CT better), volvulus, toxic megacolon, perforated viscus; recurrent imaging and want less radiation: Crohn's, ulcerative colitis, young patient; not useful in routine abdominal pain or kidney stone (poor sensitivity)
- **"ABCs"** (**A**: Air in lumen, **B**: Bones, **C**: Ca++, **S**: Soft [kidney, liver, psoas])
- **SBO**: 65–70% sensitive. SI normally contains minimal to no air, AFL = Air Fluid Level (upright film)
  - *Positive*: Multiple AFL's, loops >3 cm, "string of pearls" (air trapped in valvulae conniventes)
  - *High-grade*: > 2 AFL's, AFL's > 2.5 cm wide, or AFL's > 5 mm apart in same bowel loop.
- **LBO**: 6 cm = ULN, Cecum: 9 cm. Can perforate at 12 cm; usually has air, speckled feces, haustra
- **Free Air**: Diaphragm, double wall sign, pneumatosis, retro-peritoneal air
- **Calcification**: Stone, pancreatitis (L1/L2), aorta, spleen, phlebolith, node, fibroid, appendicolith
- **Soft Tissues**: Flank stripe, psoas borders, kidney (L1–L3), liver
- **Pneumatosis Intestinalis**: Bowel Ischemia, COPD, connective tissue disorders, enteritis, celiac disease, leukemia, amyloidosis, steroid use, chemotherapy, AIDS, idiopathic (15%)

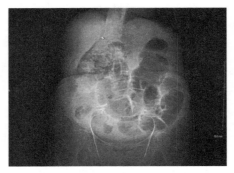

FIGURE 2.39.   Double wall sign from free air due to perforation.

THORACIC SPINE

- **Indications**: Sx > 4 wks, trauma, age < 20 or > 50, CA/weight loss, fever, IVDU, drug/alcohol abuse; immune suppression, chronic steroids, rest pain, abnormal neuro, exam neuro
- **General**: Check vertebral body heights. Cord has less room in T-spine
- **Abnormals**: Compression fractures. Bulge of the paraspinal shadow; abnormal widening of distance between pedicles (each should be slightly wider than above)

LUMBAR SPINE

- **Indications**: Sx > 4 wks, trauma, age < 20 or > 50, CA/weight loss, fever, IVDU, drug/alcohol abuse, immune suppression, chronic steroids, rest pain, abnormal neuro, exam neuro
- **Exceptions**: Suspect ankylosing spondylitis, patient insistence, litigation planned, worker's comp
- **Misses**: Transverse process fx often missed: may see psoas margin obliteration
- **Chance Fx**: Associated with MVA and lap belt. Most common at T10–L4
- **Metastases**: Usually at pedicle: best seen on AP view

GENERAL ORTHO

■ **Arthritis**: Osteoarthritis (knees, hips, spine, fingers) > rheumatoid (hands, neck), gout > other
  ● *OA*: ASYMMETRIC narrow joint space, osteophytes, sclerosis both sides, bone cysts
  ● *RA*: SYMMETRIC narrow joint space, NO osteophytes, local osteopenia, thin cortex; erosions > subluxations
  ● *Gout*: Large erosions with hook-like margins; soft tissue swelling, tophi may calcify
  ● *AVN*: ONE side of joint, Early: Patchy sclerosis, Later: Subcondral lucency
■ **Calcification**: DDx: Dermatomyositis, venous insufficiency, infection, metastases, vitamin D, scleroderma, tumoral calcinosis, heterotopic ossification, myositis ossificans
■ **Callous**: Forms in 2–6 wk post fx for adult
■ **CT Needed**: Skull, spine, pelvis, plateau, calcaneus, occult hip (MRI)
  ● *Mets*: Esp. to pedicle of spine. blastic: prostate, breast; lytic: kidney, thyroid, lung, breast
■ **Foreign Bodies (FB)**: Visible: Glass, metal except aluminum, gravel; not visible: soda-can pull tab, wood, plastic, bones, or freshwater fish
■ **Osteomyelitis**: MRI or bone scan best. Plain films: Subperiosteal elevation, swelling > lytic: 3–4 wk

ORTHO PITFALLS AND MISSES

■ **Malpractice**: Pelvis + spine: 44% > extremities: 22% > hand: 14%
■ **Misses**: Scaphoid, triquetrum, femoral neck, sacrum, acetabulum, tibial plateau; segond (tibial plateau spine avulsion), patella, calcaneus, talus, any 2nd fx
■ **Pairs**: Galeazzi = distal radius + distal radioulnar joint, often with ulnar nerve involvement; distal radius intra-articular or die-punch fracture + carpal bone; monteggia = proximal ulna + radio-capitellum dlc, often with radial nerve involvement; pelvis is a ring, often two fractures; maisonneuve = ankle + proximal fibula fractures; lumbar + calcaneus

PEDIATRICS

■ **General**: Children are more likely to have an unseen Salter-Harris type 1 fracture than a sprain
■ **Buckle Fx**: Common fx especially at the wrist. May be subtle. Also seen: humerus
■ **Greenstick**: Long bone fx where one side of cortex breaks, but other remains intact

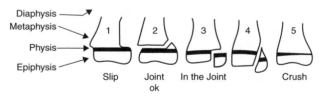

FIGURE 2.40. Severity by Salter Harris.
1 and 2: Least = extra-articular; 3 and 4: Next = intra-articular; 5: Worst = crush

UPPER EXTREMITY

Consider comparison views in equivocal cases.
■ **Shoulder**: Three views
  ● *A-C joint*: Inferior aspect of acromion and clavicle should line up
  ● *Misses*: Posterior dislocation, Pancoast tumor, lung disease, avascular necrosis, pathological fx
■ **Elbow**: Fat pad sign = occult fracture
  ● *Lines*: Anterior humeral: > one-third of capitellum should be anterior to it; radio-capitellar: Should line up dislocation present
  ● *"CRITOL" (Ossification order*: **C**apitate, **R**adial, **I**nternal epicondyle, **T**rochlea, **O**lecranon, **L**ateral epicondyle)
■ **Wrist**: Know anatomy. Check lateral view that lunate not empty. Intracarpal joint > 2 mm is abnormal
  ● *Misses*: Occult scaphoid, torus, dorsal chip fx, lunate dislocation, scapho-lunate disassociation; beware of minor radius fractures that enter joint as they often have 2nd fx or dislocation
■ **Hand**: Three views. Look carefully for small avulsion fractures at joints
  ● *Misses*: Rotation cannot be assessed on X-ray. Serious ligament injuries can be X-ray negative

LOWER EXTREMITY

■ **Pelvis**: Check each ring. Posterior acetabular line, arcuate line. Widened SI joint > 5 mm
  ● *Misses*: Acetabular fx, subtle dislocation, sacral fracture
■ **Hip**: Two views: AP pelvis + lateral hip. Adjusting exposure may help see subtle fracture
  ● *Misses*: Pubic ramus instead of hip, occult hip fracture (if can't walk, admit for MRI), impacted fx
  ● *AVN*: Early: Sclerosis starts after 2 wk. Late: Subcondral lucency
■ **Knee**: 10% of films are positive. Fat-fluid level means intra-articular fracture
  ● *Rules*: No X-ray needed if all of: Age < 55, patella and fibular head NT, can flex 90° and able to walk
  ● *Misses*: Plateau, Segond, patella (skyline view may help)
  ● *Ca++*: Chondrocalcinosis knee > wrist. DDx: pseudogout >> hypomagnesemia
■ **Ankle**: 10% +. If no fx seen but anterior + posterior effusion > 15 mm get a CT
  ● *Rules*: No X-ray needed if all of: able to walk four steps, nontender: maleoli, 5th metatarsal and navicular
  ● *Misses*: Talus, wide mortise without fracture, calcaneus
■ **Foot**
  ● *Misses*: Metatarsal stress fracture, Lisfranc fracture (look for loss or normal alignment)
  ● *Dancers Fx*: An avulsion of the peroneus brevis at the base of the 5th metatarsal; heals well
  ● *Jones Fx*: A fracture of the proximal shaft of the 5th metatarsal; heals slowly; often requires ORIF

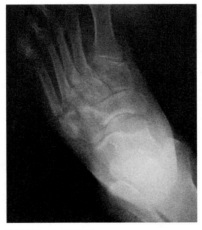

FIGURE 2.41.   Jones fracture.

■ **Calcaneus**: Normal Bohler's angle usually > 30°; CT if + fx or suspect missed fx

HISTORY OF ED ULTRASOUND
- **Opposition**: Mostly from radiology
- **Support**: AMA resolution 802, ACEP, AAEM, AHRQ (for use of guided central lines)
- **Credentials**: Done locally by each department or hospital

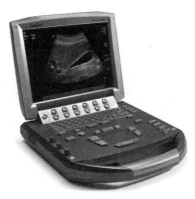

FIGURE 2.42. Bedside ultrasound machine.

BASICS
- **General**: ED US should not replace a formal study. It's an adjunct to expedited decision making
- **Probes**: Curvilinear: 2.5 megaHz. Small footprint gets between ribs. For deep structures, organs. Linear Array: 5–10 megaHz. Better resolution, less penetration: for small parts, vascular, FB
- **Marker**: Keep to patient's right side or cephalad and dot on right side of screen (except cardiac)
- **Quality**: Decreased with: obesity, PTX, PO contrast, SQ emphysema, bowel gas
- **Artifacts**: Shadow, edge artifact, reverberation, comet tail = ring down, posterior enhancement; mirror image, refraction, side lobe, aliasing, tissue vibration
- **Definitions**: Hyperechoic: Appears whiter; Hypoechoic: Appears darker gray; Anechoic: Appears black
- **Image**: Focus zone and equalizers are important
- **Document**: "I did an ED BEDSIDE LIMITED study of [organ] for [indication] and found [finding]"
- **Pitfalls**: Not visualizing entire organ, not following up on equivocal findings, no formal study done
- **Safety**: No radiation (unlike X-ray, CT, and nuclear studies). Don't leave probe on eye for > 1 min

TRAUMA: EXTENDED FOCUS ASSESSMENT WITH SONOGRAPHY IN TRAUMA (eFAST)

■ **Technique**: Do before Foley, Trendelenberg: ↑sensitivity
■ **Free Fluid**: Small < 1 cm (few need OR), Medium=1–3 cm (60% need OR), Large > 3 cm (90% need OR)
■ **Sensitivity**: ~85% if done serially. As low as 24% in some studies. Detects > 200ml (100ml for CT)
   ● *False negatives*: Gain too high, cursory exam, inferior liver tip not visualized, clotted blood
■ **Specificity**: ~95%
   ● *False positives*: Psoas/prostate can mimic fluid, vessel (check color flow)
   ● *DDx fluid*: Blood, ascites, inflammatory (ID, pancreatitis, ischemic bowel), urine, feces, physiologic
■ **Hemothorax**: US more sensitive than CXR; picks up as little as 20 ml of fluid
■ **Pneumothorax**: Scan two to three interspaces at the most anterior part of chest in the sagittal plane; 95% sensitive (CXR: 55%). normal: lung sling and comet tail artifact
   ● *False +*: Mainstem ETT, bleb, infiltrate, contusion, ARDS, atelectasis, adhesion

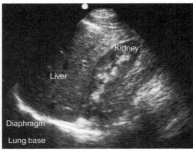

FIGURE 2.43. Normal Morrison's pouch/RUQ.
Courtesy of ERPocketbooks.com

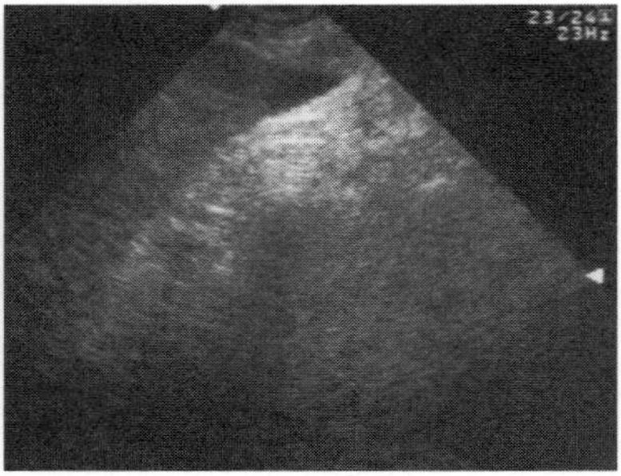

FIGURE 2.44. Small free fluid seen only at liver tip.
Courtesy of ERPocketbooks.com

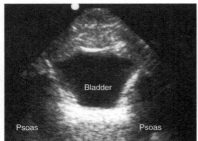

FIGURE 2.45. Normal suprapubic view.
Courtesy of ERPocketbooks.com

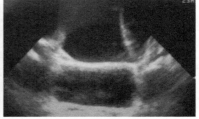

FIGURE 2.46. Large free fluid behind bladder.
Courtesy of ERPocketbooks.com

RAPID ULTRASOUND IN SHOCK AND HYPOTENSION (RUSH) PROTOCOL
■ **Basics**: Cardiac echo (see next page), IVC, eFAST for bleeding and PTX, AAA
■ **IVC**: Flat IVC is a sign of hypovolemia (mean diameter < 0.8–1cm). normal diameter is 1.6–1.75cm
  ● *Sniff test*: Full collapse: CVP <5. Some collapse: CVP = 5–10. No collapse: CVP >10. IVC check less reliable in cirrhosis, right heart failure or valve dz, all of which can dilate IVC
■ **AAA**: Retroperitoneal hematoma, Large aorta, flat IVC. Hemoperitoneum not usual (unless dead)

ECHO TECHNIQUE
↑HOB, bend knees for subcostal, LLDC position for apical 4-chamber view
■ **Effusion**: Posterior 1st (gravity), anterior alone = fatpad, no fluid at L atrium (adherent)
■ **Shock DDx**: RV dilated = PE/RVMI. RA collapse = Hypovolemia. Focal Wall Motion(apical view) = MI
  ● *PE*: Dilated RV (normal is up to 2.7 cm across), paradoxical septal movement, Distended IVC
  ● *Tamponade*: Pericardial effusion (acute < 200 cc). Right Ventricle collapse DURING DIASTOLE
  ● *Hypovolem*: Rapid small heart in hypovolemia
  ● *CHF*: Cardiogenic Shock: Dilated, hypokinetic heart
■ **Pitfalls**: Anterior only is fatpad, confusing pleural vs. pericardial fluid, PTX: can't see the heart
■ **Normals**: EF 55–70%. Septum and posterior wall 0.7–1.1 cm thick. RV chamber < 2.7 cm across
■ **Wall Motion**: Apical and Parasternal short axis view best for segmental abnormalities (MI)

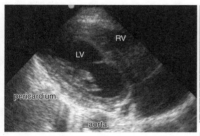

FIGURE 2.47.   Normal heart—Parasternal view.
Courtesy of ERPocketbooks.com

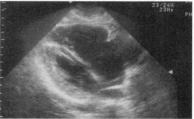

FIGURE 2.48.   Dilated RV and RA from pulmonary embolism.
Courtesy of ERPocketbooks.com

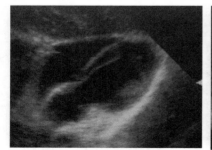

FIGURE 2.49.   Normal heart—Subxyphoid view.
Courtesy of ERPocketbooks.com

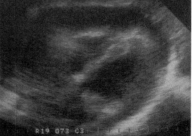

FIGURE 2.50.   Pericardial tamponade with RV collapse.
Courtesy of ERPocketbooks.com

AORTA TECHNIQUE

Measure outer wall to outer wall in transverse. View diaphragm to bifurcation.

- **Findings**: NL < 2.5 cm at diaphragm, < 2 cm at mid-aorta, < 1.8 cm at bifurcation; AAA > 3 cm (measure AP); surgery > 5 cm, rapid growth or Sx; look for clot, intimal flap
- **Tips**: Look for the aorta over spine pattern; Doppler split-screen to be certain. Dissection can be seen; start longitudinal epigastric area and try to visualize entire aorta
- **Pitfalls**: Incomplete imaging, sacular aneurysm, confusing IVC (compressible) with aorta (not); not including clots in measuring aorta diameter

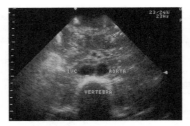

FIGURE 2.51.   Normal aorta—Transverse.
Courtesy of ERPocketbooks.com

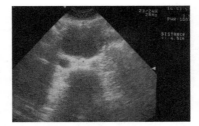

FIGURE 2.52.   4.5 cm AAA—Transverse.
Courtesy of ERPocketbooks.com

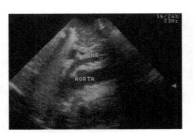

FIGURE 2.53.   Normal Aorta—Longitudinal.
Courtesy of ERPocketbooks.com

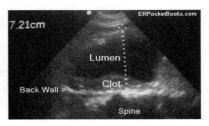

FIGURE 2.54.   7 cm AAA—Longitudinal.
Courtesy of ERPocketbooks.com

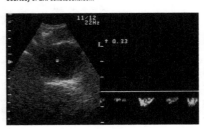

FIGURE 2.55.   Normal aorta—Transverse with doppler.
Courtesy of ERPocketbooks.com

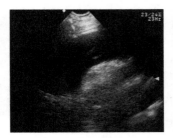

FIGURE 2.56.   Dilated aortic arch with dissection.
Courtesy of ERPocketbooks.com

GALLBLADDER

Technique: Measure bladder wall anteriorly and AP; CBD inner lumen measure

- **Gallstones**: Common: 15% of adults, therefore may be a red herring
- **Gall Bladder Wall**: Thickness: Nl < 3 mm. In acute cholecystitis, gallbladder wall is > 3 mm in 50–75% of cases
  - *DDx*: If GB wall > 4 mm consider: cholecystitis, cholangitis, hepatitis, low albumin, tumor, CHF
- **Common Bile Duct (CBD)**: Nl < 4–6 mm, 10 mm p chole, or 1 mm per decade; 33% nl in obstruction
- **Pitfalls**: Miss single stone in bladder neck; polyps don't shadow or move; confusing CBD with vessel

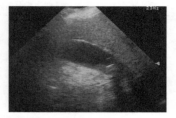

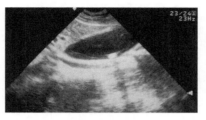

FIGURE 2.57. Gallstone in neck of gallbladder.
Courtesy of ERPocketbooks.com

FIGURE 2.58. Gallstone and pericholecystic fluid.
Courtesy of ERPocketbooks.com

KIDNEY

Technique: Left side harder: breath hold, spleen as window. Decubitus.

- **Size**: WNL: 10–12 cm; pyramids are dark; pyelo: less echogenic
- **Pain**: Stones: Hydronephrosis (see the stone: 19%); cyst > 6 cm may cause pain
- **Simple Cyst**: Criteria: Unmeasurably thin wall, fluid, no septae, anechoic, distinct, round/oval, enhancement
- **Pitfalls**: False (+) hydronephrosis: bilateral, overhydration, full bladder, pregnant, cysts, reflux

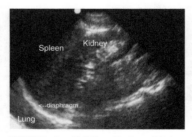

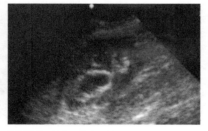

FIGURE 2.59. Normal left kidney with spleen and diaphragm.
Courtesy of ERPocketbooks.com

FIGURE 2.60. Moderate hydronephrosis.
Courtesy of ERPocketbooks.com

APPENDICITIS AND INTUSSUSCEPTION

Limitations: Worse in obese patients

- **Benefits**: No delay for contrast; no radiation, use liberally in pediatrics and obstetrics
- **Appendicitis**: In thin patients, sensitivity is up to 88%, which is close to CT at 94%. Consider using first. (+): tubular, noncompressible, > 6 mm, aperistaltic, blind-ended sac connecting to cecum
- **Intussusception**: 85%/98%. Usually > 5 cm; donut or target sign, pseudokidney sign; donut or target sign = concentric rings (hypoechoic outer ring, hyperechoic inner ring)

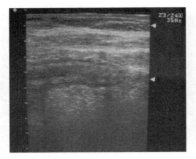

FIGURE 2.61.   Appendicitis: Longitudinal.
Courtesy of ERPocketbooks.com

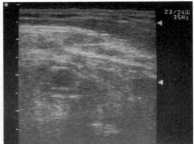

FIGURE 2.62.   Appendicitis: Cross-section.
Courtesy of ERPocketbooks.com

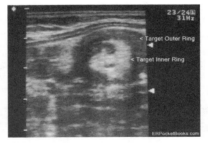

FIGURE 2.63.   Intussusception: Target sign.
Courtesy of ERPocketbooks.com

OB/GYN

Technique: Trans-abdominal first; trans-vaginal: let patient put probe in vagina herself.

- **Ectopic**: No IUP: beta < 1000-worry more, > 60,000: consider a molar pregnancy or completed abortion
- **Weeks/See**: 5–6 wks: sac; 6–7 wks: pole and cardiac motion (if present 85% go to term); Nl FHR: 90–170; if crown-rump > 5 cm, should see cardiac motion. Nl FHR: 90–170, but 120–180 if > 8 wks
- **Pseudosac**: Endometrial blood seen in < 20% of ectopics: central and fills cavity, no double ring or embryo
- **Abruption**: Placenta > 4 cm, lucent collections, particles in fluid, US only 40% sensitive
- **Vaginal Bleed**: NL endometrial stripe < 15 mm (5 mm post-menopausal); no trans-vag probe if recent procedure
- **Ovaries**: Located just medial to iliac vessels; superior and lateral to uterine fundus
- **Torsion**: Color Doppler; multiple follicles 8–12 mm in cortex of enlarged ovary (congestion); 20% §mass
- **Pitfalls**: Cornual ectopic mimicking IUP—surrounding uterine mantle < 8 cm, ignoring echoic fluid

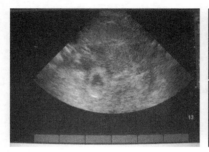

FIGURE 2.64. Ruptured ectopic with clotted blood.
Courtesy of ERPocketbooks.com

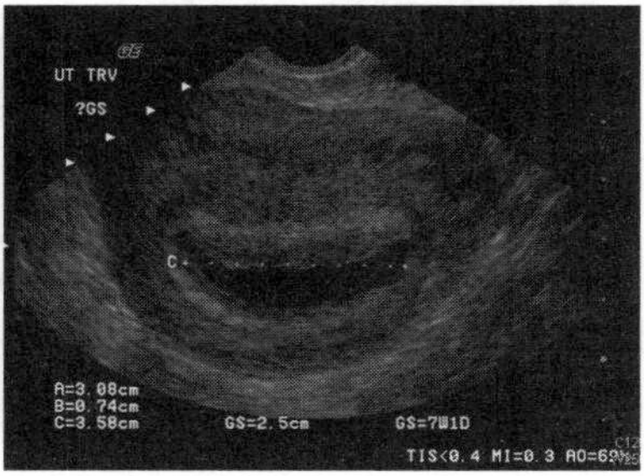

FIGURE 2.65. Pseudo-sac.
Courtesy of Julie Vajnar PA-C.

SMALL PARTS AND PROCEDURES

See Central Lines: Use of Ultrasound section on page 79

- **Probe**: Use 7.5 megaHz linear probe to visualize structure close to the surface
- **Abscess**: Appear hypoechoic or anechoic during the initial stages; later more heterogeneous; obtain images in multiple planes; identify surrounding nerves, lymphatics, and vessels; pseudoaneurysms and vessels mimic abscesses if you check only one plane; Doppler helps. Utilize contralateral limbs and adjacent areas of normal appearing tissue for comparison.
- **Foreign Bodies/Splinter**: 90–95% sensitive: echogenic with shadow or comet tails. Scanning underwater helps for small superficial objects. Leave 1cm between skin and probe; visibility: Wood > glass > plastic > metal; inflammation causes black rim of fluid (takes 2d); short angiocath "finder needle" left in place for localization or real-time guidance of forceps
- **Ophtho**: Safe, but don't press down in trauma and don't scan long or eye heats up
  - *Technique*: Eyelid closed; compare to other side
  - *Vitreous*: Retinal detachment shows intraocular white membrane. Can see lens dislocation
  - *Hematoma*: Retrobulbar hematoma can be seen as dark fluid collection
  - *Nerve*: Optic nerve sheath > 5 mm (> 4.5 mm age 1–15 yr) is an earlier sign of ↑ICP than papilledema; measurement taken 3 mm behind optic disc. Sensitivity > 95%, specificity 63%
- **Ortho**: Arthrocentesis. Comparison to other side can be quite helpful
  - *Tendon*: Can see halo of fluid around tendon in inflammatory conditions
  - *Joint*: Can see fluid in joint. Fractures may be visualized as break in cortex
- **Peds**: Appy, pyloric stenosis (diameter > 15 mm, length > 16 mm, wall thickness > 3 mm), intussusception
- **Urology**: Post-void residual urine: volume = ½ diameter cubed

VASCULAR AND DVT

(For use in central lines, see Circulation section on pages 77–80)

- **Technique**: Distend vein by frog leg and optionally, reverse Trendelenberg; may be able to see valves
- **Sites**: Limited: Common femoral at saphenous, proximal deep and superficial femoral, popliteal
- **Positive**: Noncompressibility: Most sensitive and specific; no flow augmentation with calf squeeze. Clot: Anechoic or hypoechoic and noncompressible (may be only positive finding)
- **Negative**: Chronic Clot: More echogenic than acute. (MRI if unsure). Normal: Anechoic and compressible. If negative, repeat in 3–7d to pick up false negative isolated calf vein thrombi propagation
- **Arterial**: Should have triphasic Doppler flow. Occlusions appear as echoic areas

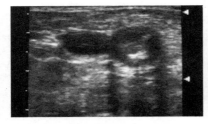

FIGURE 2.66.   Arterial thrombosis.
Courtesy of ERPocketbooks.com

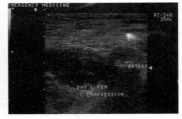

FIGURE 2.67.   Noncompressible DVT.
Courtesy of ERPocketbooks.com

CONTRAST ISSUE

■ IV Contrast

- *Dye types*: High Osmolality: All reactions = 13%, severe = 0.22%, very severe = 0.04%. Low Osmolality: All reactions = 3%, severe = 0.04%, very severe = 0.01%.

- *Utility*: Low utility unless trauma, vascular process, or very thin patient. Helps if infection or cancer; Basak et al.: 93 pts. with abdo pain had CT s̄ and c̄ Contrast helped in one, but missed one that noncontrast dx'd

- *Contraindications*: Only absolute contraindication = anaphylaxis, true iodine allergy (seafood does not count)

- *Cautions*: > 250 ml contrast volume, contrast in prior 72 hr. Renal: DM, dehydrated, CHF, RI (even dialysis patient may have residual function. Dialyze w/in 24 hr). Diseases: Pheo (HTN crisis), sickle cell (crisis), thyroid (storm), Myasthenia Gravis (exacerbation). Breast Feed: Pump and discard for 48–72 hr.

- *Minor reaction*: 3% of low osmolality, 12% of high osmolality: N, V, metallic taste, hot flash

- *Major reactions*: Seizure, hypotension, dysrhythmia, bronchospasm, anaphylactoid, renal (see topics that follow)

- *Anaphylactoid*: 0.04% (1 in 100K die): acute: Sz, BP, dysr, RAD, kidney; delayed: CPR, BP, CHF. Risk↑: Prior reaction (may do OK), asthma, any food allergy (shellfish no worse than others); beta-blocker (Epi won't work to treat). Premed: Hydrocortisone 200 mg + Benadryl 50 mg IV + ephedrine 25 mg PO 1 hr prior to CT.

- *Nephropathy*: ↑mortality, 30% permanent RI, 0.1–1% temporary dialysis, < 0.5% permanent dialysis. Timing: ↑Cr starts within 48 hr and peaks 3–5d. Usually back to nl by 7–10d. Metformin: Don't restart until assured that Cr is < 1.4 when rechecked 3–5d later. Risk↑: Kidneys: Creatinine > 1.4, GFR < 60 ml/min, proteinuria. Meds: NSAIDs, diuretics, ACEI, pressors. Diseases: Multiple myeloma, cirrhosis, HTN, CHF, DM (even with nl GFR). Other: Age > 70 yr, dehydration.

- *Nephropathy prevention*: Consider alternate or noncontrast study. Ensure adequate hydration. Use low ionic contrast. Avoid diuretics, NSAIDS, nephrotoxins, dopamine. Saline: Recommended: 0.9% NS at 1 ml/kg/hr for 24 hr. Bicarb: 3 amps sodium bicarb in 1 L D5W at 3 ml/kg/hr for 1 hr prior, then 1 ml/kg/hr for 6 hr after; N = 353 high-risk patients: 25%↓GFR in 12%/13% in saline/bicarb groups but hemodialysis in four from saline group, but only two from bicarb group (not significant). NAC: Uncertain utility: Mucomyst 600–1200 mg PO BID on day before and day of CT (four doses total).

- *Metformin*: Do not restart until renal function checked and OK at least 48–96 hr p dye (GFR at least 40)

■ Other Contrast

- *Without*: Consider unenhanced CT for fewer delays (especially if worried about AAA) and ↓risk. Consider contrast in abdo CT if: r/o appy and pain < 6 hr, CT already backed up 2 hr, skinny patient

- *Oral*: 2–3 hr to reach distal colon. Risk: Allergy, aspiration, delays, delays, delays

- *Rectal*: Best for appendicitis (not barium). Risk: Perforation, doesn't reach cecum:18%

- *Esophageal*: "B-M" (**B**arium could cause **M**ediastinitis in perforation, but inert in lung); "G-P" (**G**astrographin causes **P**neumonitis if aspirated, but not mediastinitis)

- *Other*: Consider bladder or in wound for trauma

HEAD CT

■ **Indications**: Sudden HA, abnormal exam, HA > 3 wk, HA worse with valsalva, papilledema, frequently wakens patient, concern for CVA, age > 50, not c/w primary HA, judgment.
- *Trauma*: Adult: History: Age > 60–65, Sz, EtOH, vomiting, generalized HA, auto vs. ped., fall > 3 ft, ejected.
- *Exam*: Signs of basilar, depressed or other skull fx, AMS, abnomal CNS exam. Age < 18: AMS, sign of skull fx, vomit, global HA, abnormal exam. NOT: Isolated LOC. Age < 2: unknown mechanism, scalp hematoma, AMS, fall > 3 ft

■ **Contrast**: Consider with and without contrast for metastasis (breast, lung, GI, GU), abscess, CVA, or cysts

■ **Abscess**: Hypodense + hyperdense fringe. IV contrast may help

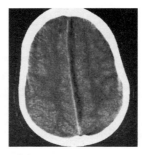

FIGURE 2.68.   Subdural empyema: A neurosurgical emergency.
Courtesy of ERPocketbooks.com

■ **Aneurysm**: SAH, but also can cause parenchymal bleed
■ **Bleed**: HTN: Basal ganglia, internal capsule > thalamus, CBL, brainstem. If heterogeneous, think tumor. CT best for acute bleed. MRI better for chronic bleed or possible cerebellar bleed.
■ **Basal Ganglia**: Globus Pallidus: Low density lesion in CO tox
■ **Calcification**: Age, ↓↑PTH, CMV, toxo, Wilson's, CO, lead, anoxia, chemo, XRT, CA, Sturge-Weber, TB, AVM, tuberous sclerosis, cystircercosis, echinococus, trichinosis.
- *Peds*: "ToRCHeS" (**TO**xoplasmosis, **R**ubella, **H**SV, **C**MV = #1, **S**yphilis)
■ **Edema**: Early: loss of blood-brain barrier.
- *DDx*: tumor, bleed, hypoxia, CVA
■ **Enhancing**: Ring Enhance.
- *DDx*: Mets, abscess, septic emboli, glioblastoma, infarct, contusion, cystircercosis, AIDS, lymphoma, toxo, demyelination, radiation necrosis, CA
■ **Hydrocephalus**: Early: temporal horn and 3rd ventricle; compressed sulci at top of brain
■ **Hygroma**: A collection of xanthochromic fluid in the dural space that may result from a tear in the arachnoid allowing CSF into the dural space or from effusions from injured vessels
■ **Metastases**: Lung, breast, GI, GU, skin > lymphoma, prostate, neuroblastoma, renal, thyroid, placenta
■ **Sinuses**: Sinusitis: air-fluid level or complete opacification is usually acute.
- *Mucous retention cyst*: Common incidental finding; usually don't need further eval. unless they are progressive, unsmooth, calcified, or are associated bony erosion
■ **Stroke**: CT often nl <12–24 h. Earliest finding is gray/white junction blurring, edema max at 3–5d
■ **Trauma**: Be systematic: Scalp, bones, AFL, sinus, orbit: Apex, rim sudural, brain, cisterns, brainstem.
- *Fracture*: Sutures > 3mm = traumatic diastasis. Orbit: Air = fx
■ **Diffuse Axonal Injury (DAI)**: Corpus callosum, gray white jxn, brainstem, basal ganglia

SOFT TISSUE NECK CT

■ **Indications:** Abscess, mass, foreign body, obstruction

■ **Contrast**: Usually use (unless foreign body). If looking at soft tissues, vascular, or masses, then use IV contrast

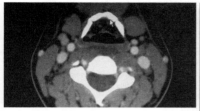

FIGURE 2.69.   Retropharangeal abscess.

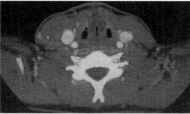

FIGURE 2.70.   Adult epiglottitis.

CERVICAL SPINE CT

■ **Indications**: Trauma, metastases/mass, cord compression when MRI or myelogram unavailable/delayed. Use when high index of suspicion despite negative plain films or if plain films positive

■ **Pros/Cons**: More sensitive than XR, but lots more radiation. Will often pick up additional fractures not seen by plain films

THORACIC AND LUMBAR SPINE CT

■ **Indications**: Trauma, metastases/mass, cord compression when MRI or myelogram unavailable/delayed

■ **Pros/Cons**: More sensitive than XR, but lots more radiation. Will often pick up additional fractures not seen by plain films

■ **MRI**: In general, should be used only if suspicion for surgical lesion. CT good for disc but need MRI for ID/CA or hematoma/bleed

CHEST CT

Don't send an unstable patient to CT. Lifetime risk of CA from radiation up to 1 in 1000 per scan

■ **Dissection**: Contrast CT best study because of speed. 95% sensitive. Noncontrast still decent if ↑Cr

■ **PE**: Sensitivity only 83%, but always improving. Consider doing venous duplex and/or D-dimer. Always ask radiologist how good the scan quality/dye timing was and how confident they are. False pos. not rare: Lymph nodes can simulate clot. More radiation to subject, but less radiation to fetus, when compared to VQ

  • *PIOPED 2 study*: Multidetector CT (most four slice) Angio: 83%/96%, excluding the 6% with poor image quality. CT only 83% sensitive for PE. If CT negative but clinical suspicion high, 40% had PE! "Additional testing is necessary when clinical probability inconsistent with the imaging results." (Stein PD, Fowler SE, Goodman LR. Multidetector computed tomography for acute pulmonary embolism. *N Engl J Med*. 2006;354(22):2317–2327.)

■ **Traumatic Rupture of The Aorta (TRA)**: Nearby hematoma is most sensitive but not specific. Specific: extravasation of dye, pseudoaneurysm, intimal flap

■ **Coronary**: Need 64 slice scanner. 5–13 mSv. 85/90 for lesions > 50%

  • *Contraindications*: Can't hold breath 15 sec, arrhythmia, known severe calcifications, prior stents

ABDOMINAL AND PELVIC CT

Don't send unstable patient to CT. Lifetime risk of CA from radiation up to 1 in 1000 per scan.

- ■ **Aneurysm**: Abdominal aortic: surgery for sx, leak, or size > 4–5 cm. Splenic: surgery for: > 2 cm or sx, pregnant, or will become so, inflammatory changes
- ■ **Appendicitis**: Ask: Was a normal appendix seen?" Noncontrast 96% sensitive: FN higher in thin patients. Appendix > 6–10 mm, wall > 3 mm, enhancement, stranding, cecal wall thickened. 3–5% missed
- ■ **Biliary Dz**: 88% sensitive. Misses small or radiolucent stones. Good for emphysematous cholecystitis
- ■ **Bladder**: Calcification: Schistosomiasis, CA, TB, amyloidosis, certain types of cystitis
- ■ **Diverticulitis**: 95–99% sensitive
- ■ **Ischemia**: 80% sensitive: Bowel wall thickening > intramural gas > portal venous gas: 13% > perforation
  - ● *Territory*: SMA: Jejunum, ileum and R colon. Emboli can be segmental.
- ■ **Nodules**: AKA incidentaloma: Large majority benign, but may be cancer so all require follow-up
  - ● *Adrenal*: Incidentaloma mostly. 2% at autopsy. DDx: pheo, CA, cyst, myelolipoma, bleed, lymphoma
    < *4 cm*: Most are benign: re-CT in 6–12 mon. Assess for hormonal activity
    > *6 cm*: 25% are CA: surgery elective. (4–6 cm: gray zone)
- ■ **Renal Stone**: > 97% sensitive. Most radiodense. Noncontrast. Vascular calcification in pelvis can be FP
- ■ **Pneumatosis Intestinalis**: Bowel ischemia, COPD, connective tissue disorders, enteritis, celiac disease, leukemia, amyloidosis, steroids, chemotherapy, AIDS, necrotizing enterocolitis, idiopathic (15%)
- ■ **Portal Air**: Bowel ischemia, SBO, barium enema, colonoscopy, necrotizing enterocolitis, diverticulitis, intra-abdominal abscesses, toxic megacolon
- ■ **Small Bowel Obstruction**: No contrast is usually better because patient may be dehydrated: 97%/90%
- ■ **Trauma**: Use IV contrast. Look for dye extravasation. For penetrating use PO contrast as well.
  - ● *Misses*: Hollow viscus, pancreas (laceration, fluid collection), diaphragm, herniation
  - ● *Bowel*: Soft Signs: Bowel wall thick, free fluid, hematoma near bowel; hard signs: extraluminal air, extravasation of contrast
  - ● *IVC*: If flat, patient is hypovolemic.
  - ● *Kidney*: Laceration, extravasation of contrast; underperfused = pedicle injury

NUCLEAR MEDICINE TESTS

NUCLEAR MEDICINE BASICS

■ **Contraindications**: Severe pulmonary HTN
■ **Radiation**: Patients emit low-level radiation for 72 hours. Routine contact unlikely to be at risk. Patient should avoid close contact with others for at least 24 hr (sleep alone).
■ **Pregnant**: Woman should urinate frequently (consider a Foley) to minimize exposure to fetus.

CARDIAC SESTAMIBI SCANS

See Exercise Stress Test section on page 23
■ **Agents**: Technicium-99, half-life = 6 hr
■ **Rest**: With pain: 90%/70% (if not in pain during injection not sensitive)
■ **Adenosine**: If can't exercise
■ **Caffeine**: Must be free of caffeine intake x 24 hr or can get false neg
■ **Exercise**: 90% sensitive; 70% specific
■ **False Negative**: Balanced multivessel disease, caffeine < 24 hr, small but unstable lesions, poor exercise; can miss 16% of stenoses > 75%. Stress: Did they walk long enough?
■ **Selection**: If CXR is normal, only 9–10% of VQ scans will be indeterminant
■ **VQ vs. CT**: VQ is half the cost, more sensitive and five times less radiation (though not for fetus) than CT scan, but, CT better if pregnant (less radiation to fetus), abnormal CXR or considering alternate Dx
■ **Interference**: V/Q scan messes up a Sestamibi so do the Sestamibi first. Bronchospasm affects VQ results so treat it first

TABLE 2.12. Pulmonary V/Q Scans
Tc-99 and Xenon, half-life = 6h
PIOPED-1: VQ results and % with PE. Can rule out PE with nl scan or low suspicion and low prob. scan

Clinical Suspicion*	Normal VQ	Low Prob. VQ	Intermed Prob. VQ	High Prob. VQ
Low	2% had PE	4% had PE	16% had PE	56% had PE
High	0% had PE	40% had PE	66% had PE	96% had PE
All	4% had PE	14% had PE	30% had PE	87% had PE

Note: To determine yours, use known risks, signs, and symptoms, CXR and EKG, likelihood of alternate dx

GI SCANS

■ **DISIDA**: AKA HIDA: 98% sensitive. Often positive when all labs are normal and US shows only stones
  ● *Normal*: Gallbladder fills in < 4 hr (most fill in < 1 hr) = acute cholecystitis ruled out
  ● *Abnormal*: Gallbladder is not visualized by 4 hr = cholecystitis
  ● *False +*: Absent gallbladder, contracted gallbladder, gallbladder filled with stones bile or sludge, poor hepatic function, or acalculus cystic duct obstruction
■ **Meckel's**: 99 mTc-pertechnetate scan to detect heterotopic gastric or pancreatic tissue
■ **Tagged RBC Scan**: For lower GI bleed. 23–97/76–95. Uses technetium. Detects bleed rates down to 0.1 ml/min
■ **Tagged WBC Scan**: For appendicitis
■ **Testicular**: Don't use. US is faster, more sensitive, and has no radiation

OTHER CARDIOVASCULAR IMAGING

ECHOCARDIOGRAM

Technique: ↑HOB, bend knees for subcostal

■ **Normals**: Up to 11 mm: septum, posterior wall. Up to 5 mm: RV free wall. Up to 42 mm: aorta

■ **Effusion**: Posterior 1st, anterior only = fat pad, none at L atrium (adherent)

■ **Tamponade**: RV collapse, acute < 200 cc; pericardiocentesis: apex #1 site, subcostal in only 12%

■ **Shock**: RV dilated = PE/RVMI; wall motion: apical view best
  ● *Volume*: Sniff and IVC collapse: complete collapse: CVP < 5. Some collapse: 5–10. None: CVP > 10

■ **Pitfalls**: Anterior only dark-space is fat pad; pericardiocentesis in wrong spot, PTX: can't see heart

■ **Stress Echo**: 76–82/84–88. Dobutamine best agent if can't exercise; good if unable to exercise or LVH. Worse if prior MI or irregular rhythm

VASCULAR ULTRASOUND

Duplex = Doppler + Ultrasound

■ **Venous**: (See Ultrasound section on pages 53–60) B mode compression best. FP/FN if prior DVT

■ **Carotid**: Check if CVA, TIA, or Bruit. If > 70% stenosis, likely candidate for carotid endarterectomy

■ **Vertebral**: Vertebrobasilar: Only 75% sensitive for stenosis. May be difficult to image

ELECTRON BEAM CT

To determine calcium score, limited by tachycardia

■ **Utility**: To determine aggressiveness of medical rx: i.e., if statins should be started for chronic CAD

■ **Score**: < 10: Low risk; 10–100: Moderate risk; 100–400: High risk; > 400: Very high risk

■ **Sensitivity**: 50–95. Fair—misses uncalcified plaques (Good for chronic plaques)

■ **Specificity**: 51–95. Poor

CORONARY CT ANGIOGRAPHY

Limited by tachycardia

■ **Basics**: Sensitivity: 86–98%. Specificity: 74–99%. To get good images requires 64 slice CT, 10s breath hold and beta-blockers to get HR< 65
  ● *Gold standard*: Conventional angiography (identified stenoses > 50% in 56% of patients)

■ **Limitations**: Tachycardia (poor gating), high calcium score (artifact), not a 64-slice scanner, dye allergy

■ **Radiation**: Same as nuclear cardiology, but in women more radiation to breasts

TABLE 2.13. Comparison of Test Characteristics for Coronary Artery
Disease Provocative Testing

Test for Coronary Disease	Sensitivity	Specificity
Exercise stress test	66%	80%
Myocardial perfusion	87%	70%
Exercise echo	80%	81%
Dobutamine echo	78%	88%

MRI IN THE ED

■ **Indications**: Cord compression and vascular conditions are the most emergent indications

- *Cord*: Suspected spinal cord compression or injury, cauda equina, epidural abscess or discitis
- *Arteries*: Suspected vascular dissection or SAH with unobtainable or equivocal LP; CT angiogram is as good or better for most arterial conditions
- *Veins*: Suspected dural sinus venous thrombosis: magnetic resonance venography (MRV); alternate: CT venography
- *Brain*: Suspected posterior fossa CVA or hemorrhage with negative CT head
- *Abdomen*: Pregnant (don't use gadolinium), peds

■ **Next Day**: Occult hip fracture, AVN, SCFE, occult scaphoid fracture

■ **Pros**: No radiation; picks up small brain lesions and spinal cord injury missed by CT. Also better for Fx

■ **Cons**: Scan lasts 10 minutes or more. Motion can distort not just one, but all of the images

■ **Contraindications**: Pacer, aneurysm clips, metal FB in eye, claustrophobia; remove any drug patches (aluminum or other metal in backing may cause burns)

■ **Contrast**: FDA boxed warning on gadolinium contrast causing nephrogenic systemic fibrosis (NSF), a life-threatening disease causing thickening and hardening of the skin and other organs. Patients with GFR< 30, or with liver disease/transplants and any level of RI, are at risk

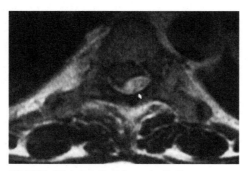

FIGURE 2.71.   MRI of spinal epidural abscess missed by CT.
Courtesy of ERPocketbooks.com

SECTION 3 ■ PROCEDURES

MNEMONIC

■ "I PREPARED" for Documentation of Procedure

Indication: What is the reason for doing the procedure?

Preparation: Sedation, ABX, analgesia (peds: sucrose, pacifier, parental holding), sterile precautions.

Risks: Discuss risks, benefits and alternatives, informed consent.

Expectation: Patient informed of what to expect including discomfort.

Positioning: Proper positioning of patient; Foley/NG tube needed?

Anesthesia: Injection of field blocks or nerve blocks; topical agents. Peds: sucrose, pacifier, parent hold.

Results: Was the procedure successful? What color fluid was obtained? Test and X-ray results.

Evaluations: Reevaluation of the patient post-procedure. Is the status improved? Neurovascular intact?

Diagnostics: Test results from lab such as CSF results, cell counts, gram stains, etc.

INFORMED CONSENT AND INFORMED REFUSAL

■ **General:** Documentation can prevent a lawsuit; should do PRIOR to procedure.

■ **Even For:** I&D and foreign body removal; consider for delayed closure of lacerations, too.

■ **Adult:** Age > 18, married, active duty with U.S. armed forces, or emancipated minor.

■ **Competent:** Able to understand nature and consequences of procedure.

■ **Risks:** Infection, scar, bleeding, damage, etc. Risks of refusal must also be explained.

■ **Benefits:** Diagnosis, treatment.

■ **Alternatives:** For example: let nature take its course, different tests or treatments and their risks.

■ **Refusals:** Should have same steps as AMA discharge; can use same form if ED has no other.

■ **Forms:** Must fill out PRIOR to procedure.

■ **DHS Info:** Must be provided for blood transfusion, breast CA, gyn and prostate exams, sterilization.

TIME OUT AND UNIVERSAL PROTOCOL

Recheck indications and contraindications.

■ **General:** Universal protocol = taking a "time out" prior to procedure to verify following five corrects: correct patient, correct site and/or side, correct equipment, correct meds, correct procedure.

■ **Indications:** Paralytics, procedural sedation, procedures. Placement of a chest-tube for pneumothorax in a nonlife-threatening situation. When MD determines correct side and does not leave the room, no further action required. If the MD leaves patient's room, he or she must mark the site with the word "YES" in indelible ink.

■ **Document:** Dictate: "Time out occurred"

POST-PROCEDURE

How tolerated, vitals, XR, lab, other studies

■ **Re-exam:** Equal breath sound for PTX, neurovascular status post reduction, vitals, etc.

■ **Imaging:** CXR for ETT and central lines.

■ **Document:** Post-procedure check and studies. **This is required for conscious sedation to be billable**.

■ **Labs:** Send body fluid for cell counts, chemistries, culture, etc.

AIRWAY

AIRWAY INDICATIONS
■ **Clinical:** Aspiration risk, going to CT scanner, combative, shock, GCS < 8, neck mass, angioedema. Expected progressive course of disease (intrafacility transport).
  ● *Caveats:* Healthy adults can have RR > 40 for days. 20% volunteers have no gag reflex.
■ **Test Based:** ABG's: pO_2 <55 on max O_2; AMS, pCO_2 >50 and pH <7.30.
  ● *Respiratory function tests:* NIF ≤ 25 (NI >60). FVC <15–20ml/kg (NI: 60ml/kg), FEV1 <10.

AIRWAY PREPARATIONS
■ **Bag Valve Mask:** Surgilube helps seal, COPD—push chest to exhale, leave dentures in.
  ● *Tough:* "BONES" (**B**eard, **O**bese, **O**bstruction, **N**o teeth, **E**lderly, **S**norer, **S**mall chin)
  ● *Assist:* Technique: hold seal and mild squeeze. When patient inhales you will FEEL the vacuum.
■ **"SOAP MIRA"**

S: Suction, McGill; Sellick too soon → vomit: wait 30 sec; succ contraindications: face fx, can't bag, shunt, eye injury, burn/crush, tox; CNS > 2d < 2 wk (MS, ALS, muscular dystrophy, CVA, cord); PNS (Guillain-Barré)

O: Oxygen by NRB even if sat = 100%; not all BVM work passively; check valve and have ready; preoxygenate with NRB x 3 min or BVM + Sellick for four huge slow breaths. Best if ↑HOB. Consider using an LMA to preoxygenate if hypoxic on NRB; this may prevent hypoxic arrest. If preoxygenated O2 sats drops 100→90 in 6min (<3 min if pulmonary dz, child or obese)

A: Airways: OP airway: size = lips to angle of jaw, nasal trumpet: size = nare to angle of jaw. Laryngoscope—three or four Mac, check light, back-up scope. Shiley and scalpel ready.

P: Pharmacology: Paralytics given rapid IV push; "LiPS" (**Li**do, **P**avulon, **S**ucc.) or "FLAVA" (**F**entanyl: 3 mcgs/kg (Blunts ICP rise), **L**idocaine: 100 mg IVP, **A**tropine (age < 5–10), **V**ecuronium (or pavulon): If prime with 1/10th dose 3 min early, get 90-sec onset; **A**midate: (= etomidate) 0.3 mg/kg)

M: Monitor and pulse ox

I: IV = running line, not infiltrated. No IV: can give succ. 2.5 mg/kg IM, 3 mg/kg for peds

R: Restraint, RT at bedside on R to pull lip

A: Assistant, inline stabilize, Sellick, BURP (back-up-right-pressure), hold tube; trumpet ready

AIRWAY BACKUPS
Anticipate difficulties
■ **Medics:** ETT: may displace: 25%, (14% medical, 37% trauma); must confirm position.
  ● *Combitube:* NG tube through and aspirate stomach before reintubation.
■ **CHF:** May die during stress of intubation. Don't defasciculate. Lie down last minute.
■ **Laryngospasm:** Smaller tube, more succ., less Sellick.
■ **Tough Airway:** Big teeth, small jaw, trauma, burn, ENT infections, CA, edema, sleep apnea. 3-3-2 rule: 3 fingers: inter-incisor, 3 fingers: chin to hyoid, 2 fingers: thyroid to jaw.
■ **Anticipate:** 2nd laryngoscope; anatomy, open mouth/dentures/sniff/crich; backups ready.
  ● *Check:* Teeth, uvula, submandibular soft tissues, ability to sniff position, mouth opening, dentures.
■ **Backup:** Have backup ready. (See Failed Airway and Back-ups section on page 73 for details.)
  ● *Options:* LMA, cart, fiberoptic, blind NT, digital intubation, crich, light wand, anesthesiologist.

TABLE 3.1.   Pretreatment Agents

Med	Dose	Onset	Good	Bad	Contras/Notes
Atropine*	0.02 mg/k	3 min	blunts ↓HR	tachycardia	minimum dose 0.1 mg
Lidocaine**	1 mg/k	3 min	blunts ↑ICP	seizure	don't push too fast or Sz
Pavulon	0.01 mg/k	3 min	defascic.	tachycardia	CBZ and phenytoin→resistance
Vecuronium	0.01 mg/k	3 min	defascic.	↑ or↑HR, BP	CBZ and phenytoin→resistance

* Atropine: Use to premedicate age < 5 (and in adults who get succ repeated or start bradycardic)
** Defasciculation: Only recommended age > 5 y

TABLE 3.2.   Induction Agents

Med	Dose	On	Off	Good	Bad	Contras/Notes
Ativan	IV 0.02–0.05/k	2–5 m	1–2 hr	safest benzo	paradoxic rxn	slow IV, titrate
Versed	IV 0.03 mg/kg	q3m	45 min	Sz, amnesia	apnea, ↑pain	decrease dose: old, + narcs
Fentanyl	IV 1–5 mcg/k	2–10 m	1/2–2 hr	↑ICP, BP	bradycardia	may get apnea before sleep
Thiopental	IV 3–5/k	30 sec	10 min	no ↑ICP	BP, RAD, RR	porphyria, BP, CAD
Etomidate	IV 0.3/k	7 sec	7 min	no ↑ICP/IOP stable BP	vomiting myoclonus	adrenal suppression—avoid repeat dosing

Note: Aspiration risk may be increased by head injury, bag-valve mask (especially if done poorly), and medications that cause vomiting (etomidate, narcotics, etc.)

TABLE 3.3.   Paralytic Agents

Med	Dose	Onset	Duration	Good	Bad	Contras/Notes
Succinyl Choline	IV 1.5–2/k. IM: 4mg/kg	50 sec	5 min	fast onset, fast offset	↑ACh: bradycardia. ↑muscle: ↑ICP/IOP ↑K: arrhythmia	difficult AW, regurgitate, burn, masseter spasm, H/o malignant hyperthermia shunt, musc. dystrophy, CVA cord, MS, GBS
Vecuronium	IV 0.2/k	3 min	30 min	nondepolarizing	long acting	L metabolism CBZ and phenytoin > resist
Pavulon	IV 0.2/k	3 min	60 min	nondepolarizing	vagolytic ↑HR	L+K metab; CBZ and phenytoin > resist
Rocuronium	IV 1mg/k	1–2 min	20 min	fast onset	long acting	L, valvular heart dz, lung dz

TABLE 3.4.   Reversal Agents

Med	Dose	On	Off	Good	Bad	Contras/Notes
Edrophonium	2–8 mg IV	5 min		reversal	bradycardia	cholinergic crisis
Neostigmine	IV 50–75 µ/k	15 min	1–2 hr	reversal	brady, V, wheeze	HR< 60, SBO, GI perf, BP < 90, BB, AMI, acidosis
Sugamadex	4 mg/kg IV	2 min		reversal	not yet approved	

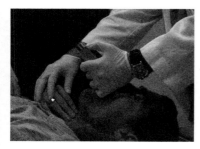

FIGURE 3.1.   Bimanual intubation.

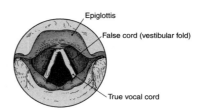

FIGURE 3.2.   Laryngoscopic view of vocal cords.
Adapted from Goldberg S, Ouellette H. *Clinical Anatomy Made Ridiculously Simple.* 3rd ed. Miami, FL: MedMaster; 2007.

Labels: Epiglottis, False cord (vestibular fold), True vocal cord

INTUBATION

■ **Acidotic:** Consider dose of bicarb 1st, because paralysis blocks respiratory compensation (avoid acidotic VT)

■ **Position:** Towel under head

■ **Tricks**
  - *Control:* Hockey-stick–shaped ETT, enter from side, pull lip to side
  - *Bimanual:* Best! Place right hand on hand of cricoid holder to adjust it
  - *Backwards Upwards Rightwards Pressure* (*BURP*): Not as good as bimanual
  - *Paraglossal:* Miller blade in to hilt then SLOWLY pull back until airway falls into view

■ **Alternate Views**
  - *10 o'clock:* Aim handle to 10 o'clock and pull.
  - *Left molar:* Insert blade from the left corner of the mouth for better view.

■ **Awake Intubation:** Usually safest choice if you think you might not be able to intubate
  - *Risks:* If not fasting much higher risk of vomiting and aspiration than with RSI
  - *Preparation:* 1. Topical: lidocaine 2 vials+1 ml phenylephrine + glycopyrolate: neb x 10 min then. 2. Sedative: Versed + fentanyl or ketamine

■ **Nasotracheal:** Must be breathing: Have backups ready, succ drawn up, crich tray, LMA, etc.
  - *Preparation*
    IV: Glycopyrolate 0.4 mg IV, Fentanyl, antiemetic.
    Neb: Glycopyrolate, 4% lidocaine, neosynephrine nasal, racemic epi.
    Nose: Lido + epi down nose, viscous on Q-tip, then on nasal trumpet. Tube bevel toward septum.
    Tube: 7.0; Endotrol tube or roll tube it to help it stay curved. Others say warm it to soften.
  - *Blind:* Advance until 10 cm left, then balloon up to center, listen for breath, neutral neck or sniff, Cricoid pressure, bevel hole medially. Depth: 26–28 cm. Tricks: Use suction cath. in Seldinger-like technique.

■ **Fiberoptic**
  - *Nasal:* Prep: lidocaine, cetacaine, dilating trumpets, antiemetic. Can advance ETT partway blind THEN put in scope and advance into trachea. Don't sedate until the scope passes or at least sees the cords. Have assistant hold scope and push in tube to 26–28 cm.
  - *Oral:* Have someone pull the tongue with a gauze or ring forceps. Preload the ETT. Advance the scope into the ringed trachea. Hold steady and advance tube.

FAILED AIRWAY AND BACK-UPS

■ Difficult Airway and Failed Airway

If sat. drops below 90%, do BVM.

- *Options*: LMA, combitube, fiberoptic, Bullar, light wand, crich, trach, digital intubation.
- *Digital*: Don't lose a finger! Comatose patient with bite blocks in. +/- stylet in "J" shape. Stand at patient's right side; index + middle finger to guide. Lots of BURP.
- *LMA*: Use if can't bag. Sniffing position, no cricoid pressure, press against posterior palate.
  Inflate with 40 ml air. Do not hold during inflation (tube should move 1 cm out during this).
  Relative Contraindications: ASP, COPD, obese, CHF; can only be used if PIPs < 20; may want to keep paralyzed to avoid aspiration.

  SIZES

1.0: Neonate	*2.5:* Age 5–9	*5.0:* Adult
1.5: Age < 1	*3.0:* Age 10+	*6.0:* Large adult
2.0: Preschool	*4.0:* Small adult	

- *Blunt neck*: Sedated awake, setup + 4% lidocaine nebulized; if see cords and cooperative > tube, if uncooperative: paralyze. If don't see cords and desat., do needle crich and to OR for a trach; smaller tube.
- *Crichothyrotomy*: Indication: mass, bleed, FBO, facial trauma, known incomplete C-spine.
  Contraindications: Can't find, age < 10: needle, larynx trauma, coagulopathy with hematoma, complete obstruction.
  How: Cut cricothyroid membrane, four fingers above sternal notch. Avoid cutting the cricoid ring. Clamp handles should face up. Extend neck, use a size 5 ET-tube or a Shiley.
  Needle: 12–14-gauge needle/catheter advanced at 45° until air withdrawn, connect to BVM. 45' max.
  Complications: 32%: bleed, dislodge, PTX, pneumomediastinum.
- *Bougie*: For difficult airway, tube change, tube confirm. > 80% success. Contraindication: failed airway.
  Technique: Shape as fishhook w/ coude tip anterior, feel for washboard effect and holdup at carina (< 40 cm). Use Seldinger technique to thread ET tube over the bougie. If it sticks, rotate ET tube.
- *Light wand*: Blind technique: load ETT, bend 90° at 12 cm from tip, paralyze, pull mandible up like drawer, stay anterior, look for cherry red glow (dull means in esophagus), pass ETT, confirm.

■ Pediatric Airways

- *Basics*: Towel under shoulder > O_2 > BVM > uncuffed tube improves view, but cuffed preferred age > 1.
- *Atropine*: Min 0.1 mg. Use to premedicate age < 5y (and in adults who get succ x2 or start bradycardic).
- *Blades*: Premie = Miller 0, term = Miller 1, 1y = Miller 1, 2y = Miller 2, 12=Mac 3.
- *ET tubes*: Cuffed tube preferred: size = 3 + years/4. In neonates use uncuffed: size = 4 + years/4.
- *LMA*

1.0: Neonate	*2.5:* Age 5–9
1.5: Age < 1	*3.0:* Age 10+
2.0: Preschool	*4.0:* Small adult

- *Needle crichothyrotomy*: Age <10y: 14-gauge IV catheter in at 45° until air withdrawn, 3.0 ETT connector to BVM. Use for 45' max. Instead of BVM can use wall O_2 at 15L/m = 50 psi. 1 sec in and 4 sec exhale.
- *Bag valve mask*: Don't bag too fast. Don't overbag (small volumes). RR=20 for a preschooler.

BREATHING

POST INTUBATION CHECKLIST
- **Depth:** 23 cm in men. 21 cm in women at mouth = 2–3 cm above carina = T3, cuffed ETT age > 7.
- **Confirm:** Basic: Direct visualization, breath sounds, tube fogging.
  - *ETCO$_2$*: Slower to change in COPD, post-arrest, and hypotension.
    False (+): vomit, carbonation, prior BVM. Make sure stays (+) for 6 full breaths.
    False (-): tracheal obstruction, adult detector used in child, no pulse.
  - *Syringe aspiration*: Can be false positive if pt. obese, CHF, drowning.
- **Bag Valve Mask:** Bag slowly until sure of ETT position and pCO$_2$. Most people bag too fast.
- **"SCAB CHANT"** (**S**oft restraints, **C**hemistry, **A**tivan prn, **B**ite block, **C**XR, **H**OB 30°, **A**BG, **N**G Tube, **T**emp)

VENTILATOR MANAGEMENT
- **Modes:** Controlled Minute Ventilation (CMV): Set rate regardless of patient effort – rarely used. Assist Control (AC): Controlled volume and backup rate, patient effort results in assisted breath. Synchronized Intermittent Mandatory Vent. (SIMV): Backup rate, patient breaths unassisted. Pressure Support (PS): Adjunct to SIMV with partial assist to patient breaths (start 10 cm H$_2$O).
- **Rates:** Starting: Assist Control of 12 or two-thirds baseline rate (prior to intubation).
  - *Special*: Neonate: 26. Peds: 20. ↑ICP: Start 14–16. COPD: Start at 10. Higher rates for acidosis.
- **Tidal Volume:** Normal Lungs: 8–10 cc/kg ideal body weight (overweight pt doesn't have bigger lungs).
- **Diseased Lung:** 6 cc/kg: can go as low as 4cc/kg with permissive hypercapnia in ARDS.
- **Peak End Expiratory Pressure (PEEP):** Start with PEEP = 5. No PEEP if head trauma or low BP.
- **O$_2$:** Prolonged O$_2$ >60% causes toxicity (usually not a problem in the ED). Try to get FiO$_2$ < 60%.
- **↑Pressures:** Keep peak (PIP) <35 and plateau <30 to avoid barotrauma. Plateau more important.
  - *Rx*: ↑HOB, pain meds, sedate, paralyze, albuterol, suction, ↑flow, bite block ↓TV: can go down to 4ml/kg; can tolerated sat down to 88%, pH as low as 7.2 and RR up to 35. Permissive hypercapnea: can ↑ICP and ↓seizure threshold. If pH < 7.2, ↑rate or give NaHCO$_3$.
- **Problems:** "DOPEGM" (**D**ynamic hyperinflation, **D**isplaced tube, **D**ehydration, **O**bstruction, **P**lug, PTX, **P**ropofol, **E**quipment, **G**I distension or abdominal compartment syndrome, **M**I)
  - *Eval*: Suction, tube OK, BVM, IVF, EKG, ABG with K, CXR (PTX may only have deep sulcus if PPV).
- **Peak Flow:** Usually 60. Use up to 120 L/min for asthma. I:E ratio from 1:2 to 1:4.
- **Barotrauma:** PTX, Pneumomediastinum, emphysema > bronchial rupture, air embolism.
  - *Causes*: ↑Volume, ↑pressure (inspiratory pause plateau best risk indicator).
- **Pneumonia:** Prevent with HOB elevation, NG tube, good cuff pressure, chlorhexidine mouth rinse.

BI-LEVEL POSITIVE AIRWAY PRESSURE (BIPAP)
- **Evidence:** Strong: CHF > COPD (resp distress or pH < 7.35 and pCO$_2$ > 45) > immune compromise.
- **Intermediate:** Asthma > pneumonia > DNR/DNI patient. Weak: Trauma, neuromuscular disease, cystic fibrosis.
- **Contraindications:** Uncooperative, apnea, FiO$_2$ requirement > 50%, AMS, aspiration risk, pulmonary fibrosis, excessive secretions, facial fracture or instability, rapid deterioration, ARDS, GI bleed.
- **Settings:** Must have at least 5cm between IPAP and EPAP. Average IPAP/EPAP: CHF: 12/6 (may start with 20/15). COPD: 13/4. RAD: 16/5. PNA: 14/6.
- **Risks:** Facial mask necrosis, gastric dilation, aspiration.
- **Tips:** If not tolerating well: start low: 8/3; different masks, pt holding mask, watch VS. ABG in 30'.

CHEST
■ Lung and Chest Wall Injuries
- *Open PTX*: Vaseline gauze taped on three sides converts it to a simple PTX.
- *Flail chest*: Analgesics, rib block, O_2 and intubate if needed. Consider splinting chest with sand bags.

■ Chest Tube
Most experts recommend never clamping a chest tube.
- *Prepare*: Conscious sedation, restraints with arm up on that side, set up with Pleurevac with suction on. Note: Never use suction initially in large PTX > 2d old as rapid re-expansion can cause ARDS and death.
- *Size*: Peds = Age + 4; Blood = 38–40 French; PTX = 28 French or smaller.
- *Position*: Arm up, prep from nipple to bed, Ancef 1 g IV, lidocaine with epi 20 cc and intercostal block.
    - 5—5th intercostal space ant. to mid axillary line (3rd if pregnant), not below nipple b/c diaphragm.
    - 4—4 cm incision (or two fingers space). A too small incision = ↑risk of tube misplacement.
    - 3—3 cm tunnel, last hole on tube at least 3 cm in. (the 10–12 cm mark at chest wall).
    - 2—2 pop through pleura with clamp, then pull it out.
    - 1—1 finger in, aim superior and anterior if air or posterior if fluid. Twist tube to release kinks.
- *Post*: 20 cm water seal, sew, Vaseline gauze, CXR. Never push tube in farther (risks infection).
- *Confirm*: Vitals and pulse-ox OK, fog in tube, meniscus moves with resps, CXR, drainage.
- *Drainage*: Thoracotomy: For bleeding > 20 ml/kg or > 3 ml/kg/h. Auto transfuse if > 500 cc blood.
- *Complications*: Re-expansion edema if lung was down for > 2d. Malposition: Hemoptysis, bleeding, shock, pressure on coronaries, etc.

■ Pneumothorax Aspiration
- *If small*: If lung apex to cupola < 3 cm, observe 3–6 hr and repeat CXR. If not worse, send home with rx.
- *Site*: 4th–5th intercostal space in anterior axillary line. Thought to be safer than 2nd ICS.
- *Catheter*: 16-gauge needle above rib margin aimed 60° cephalad then Seldinger and 8-French catheter.
- *Aspirate*: Attached a three-way stopcock and use a 50-ml syringe to aspirate; success 50–70%.
- *Observe*: Observe 6 hr and repeat CXR. If no PTX, send home. If PTX recurs, reaspirate and 6 hr obs.
- *Dispo*: Home: If PTX resolves, remove catheter and send home; may consider home with Heimlich.
- *Admit*: If PTX persists, Heimlich valve or chest tube and admit.

■ Thoracentesis
- *Contraindications*: Blood thinner, low platelets, unco-op, coughing/sneezing uncontrollably.
- *Preparation*: Decubitus film, US localization, percuss out, mark which side (L or R) in pen; US guidance decreases risk of PTX, especially in ventilated patient.
- *Technique*: Seated or supine; posterior, 5–10 cm from spine, above rib; remove 1–2 L max.
- *Post*: CXR; Lab: pH, gram stain, LDH, albumin, protein.
- *Exudate*: WBC > 1000, LDH > 200 or > 2/3 upper limit of normal, or fluid protein/serum protein > 0.5 or fluid LDH serum LDH > 0.6.
- *Complications*: PTX (if hit lung), bleeding, liver or spleen injury, air embolus, reexpansion edema (if > 1–2 L).

■ Thoracotomy
- *Indications*: Penetrating and VS in field, blunt and VS in ED (also consider for: lightning strike, hypothermia).
- *Position*: Arm up, towel under chest, intubate first, T-berg to avoid AGE; should get a R chest tube too.
- *Technique*: Cut from sternum to axilla below nipple in curve (avoid lung), then scissors, rib-spreader; retract lung, open pericardium anteriorly = medial, pump heart five times. Check for: Blood in pericardium; empty heart; air in coronaries (aspirate LV). Cardiac motion.
- *Saurbruch*: If heart moving, occlude the IVC and SVC to induce V-fib; easier to sew if less motion.
- *Repair*: Finger over wound or Foley, apical stay suture then horizontal mattress, or cardiac staples.
- *Lines*: Can place a cardiac line or give blood and meds into LV apex (avoid coronary vessels).
- *Cross-clamp*: Tear pleura, cross clamp aorta.
- *Defibrillation*: Make sure heart is full first; intracardiac paddles: Defib 15 J > 30 J.
- *Air embolism*: See air in coronaries (Rx: Aspirate LV) or hear hilar leak with each BVM (Rx: Clamp hilum).

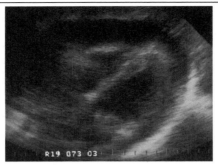

FIGURE 3.3.   Pericardial tamponade.
Courtesy of ERPocketbooks.com

■ **Pericardiosentesis**
- *Indication*: Tamponade with low BP, can't Echo (chest tube first for HTX).
- *Preparation*: Bedside Echo; thin central line kit: Seldinger or spinal needle; 18-gauge 15 cm + cath-over-needle with three-way stopcock on 30 cc syringe; sterile, lidocaine.
- *Position*: Patient sit at 30°; L of xyphoid aim at L shoulder vs. scapula, 15–45° from skin. When ultrasound guided, apex is usually the best site (subcostal best in only 12%).
- *Pitfalls*: Alligator EKG lead (misleading: ST elevation or PVCs if touch heart); FN: clotted blood.

CIRCULATION

PERIPHERAL IV TRICKS
- **Dilation:** Warm towels, arm in dependent position, NTG paste, ice on vein.
- **Tourniquet:** Use BP cuff; use two tourniquets, one above and one below.
- **Localize:** US, transillumination. Try an EJ or deep Basilic vein (it's just below brachial artery).
- **SQ Fluids:** If can't find a vein in elderly, consider hypodermoclysis: give fluids SQ using 1/2NS.

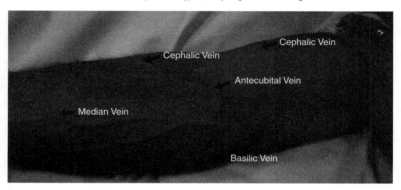

FIGURE 3.4.   Veins of the arm.

PEDIATRIC VASCULAR ACCESS
- **Illumination:** Use a transilluminator to help visualize veins
- **Umbilical:** Up to age 7 days: Cut cord at 2 cm, purse string suture; 4 French in vein 4 cm (deeper hits liver)
- **Central Line:** Subclavian or femoral; usually use size 4 French
- **Cutdown:** Saphenous: 2 cm anterior and superior to med. maleolus
- **AC Fossa:** Just lateral of midline at distal flexor elbow crease

ULTRASOUND FOR PERIPHERAL IVs
- **Preparation:** Apply a tourniquet proximally; use a high-frequency 7.5 to 10 MHz linear array transducer. Apply ultrasound gel to improve the acoustic interface. If little subcutaneous fat, use a standoff pad (can improvise with 100–250 ml bag of saline).
- **Localizing:** Arteries have thicker walls than veins, don't collapse, and are pulsatile. Veins have thinner walls, are not pulsatile. and collapse easily under pressure. If you don't see a vein where one should be, reduce the pressure of the probe on the skin.
- **Mapping:** Visualize vein in both longitudinal and transverse orientations and look for bifurcations. Note depth and make sure you have a long enough angiocath if deeper than 1.5cm.
- **Techniques**
  - *Static*: Mark the skin over the vein on both sides of your planned entry point. Use a sterile surgical pen or pressure from the round opening of the angiocath cover; can use other hand to pin vein rather than to hold the US probe.
  - *Dynamic*: Use sterile US gel and prep the US probe in a sterile fashion. Needle position may be inferred by ring down, soft tissue movement, and tenting of the vein wall.

CENTRAL LINES: BASICS

■ **Indications**
- *Absolute*: Need CVP, hypotension despite fluids, pressors, dialysis, etc.
- *Relative*: Can't get peripheral line or EJ; consider IO line instead of central line in this case.

■ **Preparation:** T-berg for high lines; towel behind back can make subclavian Tougher. Need restraints? Side: Right: Better for IJ and subclavian unless contralateral PTX; never try bilateral subclavian. US: Good for IJ and femoral, more difficult for subclavian.

■ **Site Choice:** Good: IJ with US or subclavian without: lower risk of DVT and infection. Femoral if patient can't Trendelenberg or CPR/intubating or in extremis. Avoid: Extremity with h/o prior DVT. Bilateral attempts (bilateral PTX). Femoral if need CVP. Don't go ipsilateral to pacer or vascular issue nor opposite of PTX or lung insult.

■ **Femoral:** Pros: Fast, compressible, pacer/AICD. Cons: ↑DVT, ↑ID, most comps, no CVP. How: Reverse Tberg, (abduct and externally rotate leg). Go medial to artery.
- *Pulseless*: Use US, 6 cm from pubis, or "V" method: thumb on symphysis edge, index on ASIS, go at "V."

■ **Subclavian:** Pros: Least DVT and ID, ipsilateral to PTX. Cons: COPD, hypoxia, pacer/AICD (left side).
- *How*: Right side preferred (lower lung apex), T-berg, head away. Enter at medial clavicle. Aim superior to suprasternal notch. Bevel inferior and occlude IJ with finger in supraclavicular fossa prevents wire going into EJ/IJ.
- *Supraclavicular approach*: Out of the way (CPR/trauma). Right side preferred.

  Head midline. Enter 1 cm lateral to clavicular head of SCM muscle and 1cm posterior to clavicle. Aim 45° from clavicle, 15° up from horizontal and just caudal to contralateral nipple; 2–3 cm deep.

■ **Internal Jugular:** Pros: Best for using US. Low DVT and ID. Cons: Bruit, obese, short neck, pacer/AICD (left).
- *How*: Right side preferred because right IJ usually larger and straight shot to right atrium; Trendelenberg, turning head away > 40° tends to increase overlap of IJ and carotid. Enter at apex of SCM muscle, lateral to carotid, 30°, aim at ipsilateral nipple, u < 1.5 cm deep.

■ **The Wire:** A skin incision that's too small can make it harder to feel for inappropriate sliding friction. Keep needle hub covered to prevent fatal air embolism. Don't "sink" the wire because it may enter the right ventricle and cause arrhythmias. If seems stuck, can try twisting wire, which may free up the "J" if it's stuck on a valve. Never use dilator unless sure wire in vein: no sliding friction + check wire location with US.

■ **Tricks:** Finder needle, finger on hub and patient hold breath, bevel with numbers, turn 90° for wire insertion. Have patient "hum." This works like Valsalva, but may be easier to teach.

■ **Depths:** Right-IJ: 11 cm. Left-IJ: 13 cm. Right-subclavian: 13 cm. Left-subclavian: 15 cm.

■ **Post:** Confirmation: Flows, CXR: Tip well above R atrium in SVC, no PTX, CVP reading.
- *Charting*: "SCUBA" (**S**ite and why, **C**hlorhexidine prep, **U**S use, **B**arriers, **A**ntibiotic-coated cath)
- *CVP*: WNL: 8–12cm H2O - trend more important than actual value. Give IVF until CVP > 8 or until 12–15 if on ventilator or h/o diastolic dysfunction. Bad Read: ↑Intrathoracic pressure, reference point error, tip malposition/obstruction/air bubble, ventilator.
- *Swan-Ganz*: Normal pressures are: RA: 0–6. RV: 15–25/0–6. PA: 15–25/4–13. Wedge: 4–13.

■ **Complications:** > 15% overall: ID > DVT > PTX, HTX, hematoma (confirm wire in), arterial injury, air embolism, dysrhythmia (don't sink the wire too deep), AV fistula, tamponade, brachial plexus.
- *ID*: Cx blood x 3 (1 from line) + tip if removed; Vanco + Gent + (Amphotericin).
- *Clotted*: Cath flow: this is a special 2 mg dose of tPA: leave in 30 min, then aspirate; may repeat x 1.

CENTRAL LINES: USE OF ULTRASOUND

- ■ **Why:** Proven safer, strongly recommended by the AHRQ, fewer complications. 15% IJ's in an aberrant location, fewer attempts, plus you can bill for use of US. Adjusting neck turn can decrease overlap between IJ and carotid artery. Can perform without Trendelenberg if necessary.
- ■ **Sites:** IJ and femoral good.
  - *Basilic vein:* Need a long angiocath. Can use the 2" catheter in central line kit. Harder to use with subclavian.
- ■ **Methods:** Localization: Find vein, check patency, choose side, pen-mark skin surface. Guidance: using US in real time during puncture.
- ■ **Technique**
  - *Screen:* Start by checking anatomy on both sides to choose best location.
  - *Set-up:* Machine in the direction you are facing. Needle tip most echogenic.
  - *Left/right check:* Touch each side of probe with your finger while watching screen.
  - *Touch:* Keep ulnar edge of hand holding transducer in contact with patient to prevent sliding.
  - *Needle angle:* Start closer to vertical so can see needle better. Once in vein, level off.
  - *Poking technique:* Hard to see needle, but see movement of soft tissues.
  - *Lidocaine injection:* Advance the needle under direct visualization injecting as you go. This achieves additional anesthesia (entering the vessel can hurt) and allows better visibility for tracking the needle tip. Be careful not to inject air because even the small bubble at the end of the syringe can completely obliterate your view.
  - *Entry:* Needle tip indents wall of the vein prior to entry. Avoid going through back of vein.
- ■ **Pitfalls:** Looking at shaft, but tip elsewhere; compressing vein so it can't be seen; left/right confusion; injecting bubbles.

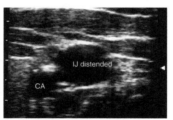

CA = Cartoid Artery; IJ = Internal Jugular

FIGURE 3.5.   Ultrasound view of jugular vein anatomy.
Courtesy of ERPocketbooks.com

INTRAOSSEOUS LINES

Check out www.vidacare.com for an instructional video in EZ-IO.

- ■ **General:** Works even in CPR: flush line after drug. Can use blood for T and C, chem, but not CBC.
- ■ **Indication:** Peds (#1 choice after peripheral IV). Can do two IOs if necessary. Safer and less painful than central line for peds and adults.
- ■ **Contraindications:** Can't identify proper site, local infection, fracture proximal to site.
- ■ **Preparation:** Sterile; give IM ketamine first if child too awake.
- ■ **Ped Sites:** Proximal tibia 2 cm distal and 1 cm medial to tuberosity on flat part of bone.
  - *Alternate sites:* Distal tibia (#1: adults) > distal femur (↑flow rates).
- ■ **Adult Sites:** Proximal or distal tibia, humerus: lateral part of greater tuberosity (put patient's hand on umbilicus).
- ■ **Technique:** Sterile (lidocaine) prep, (can put needle through gauze 2x2's dressing), (scalpel to bone), aim away from growth plate. Often hits back wall so once in, pull back 2–3 mm. Don't wiggle.
- ■ **Post:** Flush with 2 ml lidocaine, then saline, check for extravasation, protect, leg board, X-ray. IV pump may not work, may need to push with syringe or use pressure bag.
- ■ **Complications:** Through back wall > clogs (flush) > compartment syndrome, extravasation, fat embolus, Fx, ID.

VENOUS CUTDOWN

■ **Indication:** Need for vascular access; contraindicated in injured extremity.

■ **Site:** Saphenous vein 1 cm anterior and 1 cm superior to the medial malleolus.

■ **Preparation:** Betadine or chlorhexidine. Externally rotate foot; tourniquet is optional; lidocaine anesthesia.

■ **Technique:** Cut a 2.5-cm transverse incision over the vein. Blunt dissect parallel to vein with hemostat. Elevate vein. Pass two ties under the vein: one proximally, one distally. Ligate distally and use the free ends of suture for traction. With scalpel, perform small transverse incision in vein, being careful not to injure the back wall. Introduce IV catheter (without needle) through incision; secure it with the proximal tie. Suture close the skin incision and place a sterile dressing.

■ **Complications:** False passage, hemorrhage, air embolus, thrombosis, ID, transection of nerve or artery.

NG TUBES

Only 42% Sensitive for GI Bleed

- ■ **Indications:** Bowel obstruction, esp. if severe or persistent vomiting; aspiration for blood.
- ■ **Contraindications:** Relative: Mild or partial obstruction, ileus, recent facial trauma, coagulopathy.
  - • *Bariatric:* Gastric bypass: avoid blind NG, or call surgeon first.
  - • *Varices:* OK if active bleed, but not if recent bleed or recent banding/treatment.
- ■ **Anesthesia:** 4 ml of 10% lidocaine from crash cart nebulized or lidocaine spray, then jelly sniff and swallow.
- ■ **Technique:** If replacing switch nares; sitting position best. Measure for depth: Nose to ear to xyphoid. Glass of water and straw for awake patient to swallow during insertion. Coughing = malposition.
- ■ **Confirm:** Before charcoal or irrigating, confirm position with CXR or aspiration of material with pH < 4. If patient intubated or comatose, cannot rely on exam. Auscultation not reliable.
- ■ **Residual:** > 300 cc 4 hr p meal is diagnostic of gastric outlet obstruction.
- ■ **Complications:** Bleeding, perforation, vomiting, ectopic (in lungs: hypoxia. In esophagus: ↑ risk for aspiration)
- ■ **Peds:** Sizes: NG = 2 x ETT size; residual volume > 5 ml is 94% specific for pyloric stenosis.

G-TUBES

- ■ **Maturity:** Age < 1 wk: if out leave out, admit (ABX). 1–6 wk: Call GI for advice. > 6 wk = mature.
- ■ **Replacing:** Surgilube and slow steady pressure. ASAP because hole may constrict. Foley can temporize.
- ■ **Complications:** Occlusion: irrigate > declog > replace; local infection: Rx = H_2O_2. Leak: Rx = reglan, ↓rate.

PARACENTESIS

Safest with US guidance

- ■ **Indications:** Diagnostic: New ascites, r/o infected ascites. Therapeutic: Tense ascites, respiratory distress
- ■ **Contraindications:** Uncooperative patient, scar or cellulitis at site, bowel obstruction, pregnant, DIC, tPA use
  - • *Relative:* INR > 1.5–5.0 (most experts say OK at any INR—correcting more dangerous?), platelets < 50
- ■ **Preparation:** Decompress bladder, position HOB at 45–60 (bowel floats) then use US to find best pocket
  - • *Ultrasound:* Position first, use curved probe, find biggest fluid pocket with no vessels or organs in way.
- ■ **Site:** 2 cm below navel, RLQ or LLQ. Don't reposition p US. Avoid: Scars, rectus, veins, spleen
  - • *Z-puncture:* Pull skin down 2 cm before inserting needle to minimize leakage from site afterwards
- ■ **Tricks:** Put syringe on the 3-way and fill w/ fluid—use to float off any sucked in intestine if flow blocked
- ■ **Tests:** SBP: > 250 PMN > 1000 WBC. If bloody subtract 1 WBC per 250 RBC. Put 10 ml fluid in BCx bottles
  - • *Exudative:* Protein > 3 or ratio > 0.5. LDH > 200 or ratio > 0.6, Serum-Ascitic Albumin Gradient < 1.1
  - • *Other:* Glucose < 50, protein > 1 or LDH > 200 suggest secondary peritonitis. TG > 200: chylous

DIAGNOSTIC PERITONEAL LAVAGE (DPL)

- ■ **Contraindications:** Known penetration, need laparotomy (relative: previous surgery, pregnant, ascites/cirrhosis).
- ■ **Preparation:** NG tube, Foley, betadine, lido with epi; closed—fast and solo; open—old scar, pregnant.
- ■ **Open:** 11 blade 2 cm below navel (except pelvic fracture or pregnant) >18 gauge 45° down.
- ■ **Closed:** Use Seldinger technique.
- ■ **Lavage:** 10 ml/kg or 1 L warm LR, wait 5 min, then slosh and take out > 300 cc.
- ■ **Positive:** RBC: Blunt: 100 K RBC, penetrating: 5–50 K RBC or 5–10 cc frank blood. WBC: Blunt: 500 WBC; penetrating: 200 WBC; Other: Amylase > 175, vegetable matter.
- ■ **Limitations:** Too sensitive = too many negative exploratory laparotomies; misses retroperitoneum.

CYSTOGRAMS AND URETHROGRAMS

■ **Cystogram:** KUB then 100 ml contrast via Foley then repeat KUB, then 200–300 ml more contrast, then multiple views, then drain and do a final KUB.

■ **Retrograde UrethroGram (RUG):** Insert Foley 2 cm only without lube then 1 cc water in balloon, the penis to side. No filling = complete tear.

FORESKIN PROCEDURES

■ **Entrapped Foreskin:** Cut zipper mechanism with wire cutter to avoid second trauma from unzipping.

■ **Paraphimosis:** A urologic emergency: necrosis can result from edema. Many methods to reduce follow and pretreating with lidocaine gel may help.

- *Digital*: Place index fingers on the dorsal border of penis and the thumbs on the end of the glans. Push the glans back through the prepuce with the help of constant thumb pressure.
- *Ice*: Put in a glove full of ice for 5 minutes before manual reduction effective in 90% of patients.
- *ACE wrap*: Starting from the glans ending at the base of the penis for 5–7 minutes.
- *Osmotic*: Wrap in gauze soaked in 50cc of 50% dextrose for an hour can help reduce edema.
- *Puncture*: Puncture the foreskin in multiple areas to allow edematous fluid to escape during reduction.
- *Aspiration*: Use a 20-gauge needle parallel to urethra to aspirate 3–12 ml blood from glans, then reduce.
- *Vertical incision*: Place 2 straight hemostats at 12:00 position for hemostasis. Next incise with a longitudinal incision (1–2 cm). After reduction, suture margins.

■ **Priapism**

Corpus Cavernosum Aspiration

- *Preparation*: Meds (Sudafed, narcotics, IV fluids), sterile prep and drape.
- *Anesthesia*: Penile block = circumferential infiltration of 1% lidocaine.
- *Technique*: 19-gauge butterfly in lateral midshaft of both corpi. Aspirate/milk shaft until blood becomes redder; then inject 1:10,000 epinephrine or neosynephrine (except if on MAOI or h/o CAD/CVA).
- *Observation*: Observe for 2 hr post-procedure for side effects or reoccurrence.

VAGINAL DELIVERY: CALL OB, NICU

- **Bimanual:** Contraindicated if bleeding. Check for cord, presenting part. When cervix is 10 cm, push.
- **Fetal Monitor:** Toco: top = fundus, zero it, UC? Nonstress test: OK: 2 x 15 bpm rise > 15 sec in 20 min.
  - *WNL*: HR variability > 5; HR: 120–160 if > 20 wk (> 160: Pitocin, ID, F, tox, O_2); OK: accel. and early decel.
  - *Early decel*: Skull pressure with contraction > ↑vagal tone, HR > 100.
  - *Variables*: Cord, severe ≥ 60 sec; Rx as previous + elevate presenting part, reverse T-berg.
  - *Late decel*: Placenta; 80% born OK; start + end p UC. Severe: drop > 45 bpm or lasts > 30 sec. Rx: LLDC, IVF, O_2 by FM, Mg, stop Pitocin, check pH, cord?
- **Delivery:** If bulging perineum, can see presenting part, prepare for ED delivery. Call OB and NICU. IVF and O_2 and fetal monitor. Betadine perineum; Ritgen's maneuver, suction nose then mouth once head out. Check for nuchal cord. Gently guide head down until anterior shoulder out then guide up. Once out, suction again. Clamp and cut cord. Stimulate and dry infant. Cord gas.
- **Breech:** Cord prolapse: hand in vagina to elevate presenting part, C-section.
- **Dystocia:** 1% of deliveries; have patient stop pushing. Call for help—you have 5 min to save baby.
  - *Maneuvers*: McRoberts (knees to chest), suprapubic pressure, down, Wood screw, procto-episiotomy, free post arm, break clavicle (outward to avoid PTX).
  - *Zavanelli*: Rotate fetal head into occiput anterior position and push back in and do C-section.
- **Episiotomy:** Indications: tearing. Perform in midline posterior with Mayo scissors.
- **Placenta:** Should deliver w/in 30 min. Massage uterus, but don't pull cord. Examine for missing chunks.
- **Hemorrhage:** > 500 ml EBL. Early: 0–24 hr post-partum. Causes: atony, retained products, laceration, DIC.
  - *Rx*: Uterine massage, Pitocin 40 u/1L, search for and remove retained products. Sew lacerations. 2nd Line: Pack uterus, Methergine 0.2 mg IM q2–4h > Hemabate 0.25 mg IM q15–90m > embolize > OR.

CRASH ED CESARIAN SECTION

- **Indication:** > 24 wks, no response to 4 min of resuscitation. Do not do prearrest.
- **Preparation:** Be sure > 24 wks so baby viable. Call NICU + OB, place Foley. Resuscitate for 4 min, baby out in fifth min.
- **Procedure:** Cut symphisis to umbilicus, bladder down, cut uterus low, scissors.
- **Post:** Continue resuscitation attempts: mother's hemodynamics may improve once baby delivered.
- **Outcome:** If completed in < 5min, > 90% of babies survive neurologically intact.

CENTRAL NERVOUS SYSTEM

LUMBAR PUNCTURE

- **Contraindications:** Coagulopathy, mass, shock, ↑ICP, unstable airway, cellulitis over site. If severe AMS, do not LP, just treat and LP in a few days (herniate).
- **Preparation:** CBC, PT/PTT, CT, neurologic exam with fundi. Make sure well hydrated.
  - *CT 1st:* Hx: Age > 60, immune suppression, h/o CNS dz, Sz, ALOC, sinusitis, OM. Exam: Unreliable (Peds, AMS), field cut, gaze preference, leg drift; papilledema; ↓ platelets.
- **Positioning:** Three common options are used for adults and one for infants
  - *Side position:* Pro: Can do opening pressure, patient comfort (pillow between knees).
  - *Sitting:* Pro: Possibly less apnea in neonates/infants, may be easier.
  - *Hugging:* Parent on stool facing child who wraps arms around parent's neck. Pillow inbetween parent and child to round child's back. Assistant backs up the process.
  - *Baby:* Holder should make "C" with thumbs and fingers. Gather elbows to knees. If held too tightly can die from suffocation. Keep pulse ox on and watch assistant.
- **Technique:** L4–5 = interiliac crest line. Feel L3–4 and L4–5 and use larger interspace. Aim at navel. Top of interspace, keep needle and bevel parallel to spine, look from side to check angle. Use noncutting (Gertie-Marx or Whittaker) needle to minimize post-LP headache. Leg pain/paresthesia usually transient and mean the needle tip is in CSF space.
- **Pressure:** Nl: 7–18. Straining can artificially elevate. Obesity may cause higher pressures (up to 25).
  - *Low:* Dehydration, CSF leak.
  - *High:* Venous sinus clot, mass, ID, CHF, SVC syndrome, SAH,↑ pCO_2,↑BUN, pseudotumor.
  - *Rx:* Therapeutic for pseudotumor: closing pressure should be < 30.
  - *Queckenstedt's Test:* After checking opening pressure have assistant softly compress both jugular veins. Pressure should rise rapidly. If not there is spinal stenosis, cord compression or mass.
- **Post:** Rub tissue planes. Wait for gram stain results. Avoid NSAIDs because may make a blood patch ineffective.
- **Complications:** Headache, meningitis, spinal epidural abscess, spinal epidural hematoma, herniation.
  - *Post LP headache:* 4–40%. Young women at highest risk. Preventing: Use smaller needle, use noncutting (Gertie-Marx or Whittaker) needle, lie prone afterwards.

VP SHUNT TAP

- **Indications:** R/O shunt infection: 90% occur within 6 mon of revision. Sx of shunt infection include F, AMS, V, abdo pain, shunt malfunction > meningeal signs.
- **Contraindications:** Inexperience, skin infection over reservoir. Always discuss with neurosurgeon first.
- **LP Instead:** OK to do. May not pick up early infection, ventriculitis, or infection confined to shunt.
- **Preparation:** Trim hair. Meticulous sterile precautions. Make sure betadine dries at least 2 min. Patient should be prone, supine, or decubitus. Use LP tray with added supplies noted in the "Technique" section here.
- **Technique:** Nick skin with 18-gauge, then use 25-gauge butterfly to access at 30° angle to skin. 30° avoids damaging floor of reservoir. Don't aspirate. Fluid should drain passively. Measure pressure. Remove only 4–6 ml of CSF.
- **Complications:** Shunt damage, shunt infection.

CEREBROSPINAL FLUID (CSF)

Caution! No CSF test can reliably differentiate viral vs. bacterial!

- **RBCs:** RBC tube 4: >100 is abnormal. SAH: Less sensitive < 12 hr.
  - *Crenation*: Present if RBCs are old, but ?reliability, brief delay to lab might cause.
  - *Xanthochromia*: 60% at 6 hr, 90% at 12 hr.
  - *DDx*: RBC, bilirubin, dietary carotenoids.
  - *CSF D-dimer*: Should be (+) in SAH and (-) in a traumatic tap (uncertain validity).
- **WBCs:** Normal< 5 WBCs/hpf (neonate < 30) BUT worry if any WBCs and AIDS, ↓ immunity, any PMNs at all, partial Rx'ed, sick.
  - *Traumatic*: Traumatic tap: 1 WBC per 500 RBC is what you'd expect, but it's actually 1 WBC:5000 RBC. It's much safer to just ignore the calculation. If WBCs are high, worry even if traumatic.
  - *Monos*: Viral, fungal (100–500), Guillain-Barré.
  - *PMNs*: Early viral/fungal, IVIG, bacterial (1–1000 WBCs, > 80% PMN—but not always).
  - *Lymphs*: < 20% PMN is usually viral (u 10–1000 WBC) BUT CAN BE NONVIRAL.
- **DDx**
  - *Viral*: West Nile, coxsackie, echo, arboviral, HSV, HIV.
  - *Bacterial*: Early bacterial (10% of bacterial), partially treated bacterial; also: listeria, syphilis, rickettsia, leptospirosis, Lyme.
  - *Fungoid*: Crypto, cocci, TB (100–500 WBC).
  - *Other*: Endocarditis, Guillain-Barré, cancer.
- **Glucose:** NI: 50–80; viral ID: nl; bacterial ID: < 50 or < 40% serum; fungal/TB: low, < 40.
- **Protein:** NI: 20–45; viral ID: < 100; bacterial ID: > 150–220; fungal/TB > 100.
  - ↑*Protein DDx*: ID, trauma, SAH, endocrine, tox (alcohols, metal, dilantin), MS/GB, CNS thrombosis, CA, CVA.
- **Gram Stain:** 50–80/90; antigen panel (CSF, urine, blood) only if partially rx'd, ↓ immunity.
- **Neonate:** < 2 wk: WBC up to 25–30 and protein up to 170 OK, glucose 30–115.
- **Other Tests**
  - *Bacterial*: Latex agglutination: 66%, VDRL, RPR/FTA, lactate: nl < 35, Lyme IgG + IgM.
  - *Viral*: HIV, HSV + VZV PCR, Coxsackie titers (coxsackie, echo, cocci), West Nile titer.
  - *Fungal*: AFB, CrAg: 90% sensitive, India ink: 50% sensitive, fungal culture.

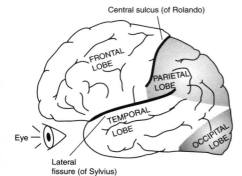

FIGURE 3.6. The brain.
Adapted from Goldberg S, Ouellette H. *Clinical Anatomy Made Ridiculously Simple.* 3rd ed. Miami, FL: MedMaster; 2007.

EYES

■ **Anesthesia:** Proparacain doesn't need refrigeration, stings less and starts working faster.
■ **Lateral Canthotomy**
  ● *Anesthesia*: Inject lidocaine with epinephrine into the lateral canthus.
  ● *Hemostat*: Crush skin at lateral canthus for 1 min + with hemostatsis and to mark area.
  ● *Scissors*: Cut the lateral canthus down to the orbital rim (usually 1–2 cm deep). Cut and release the inferior crus of the lateral canthal tendon (avoid globe).
  ● *Tonopen*: Remeasure IOP. If < 30, stop. If > 40, cut the superior crus from orbital rim.

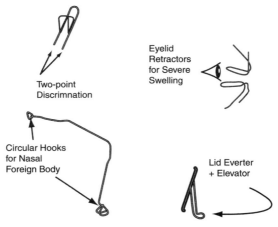

Two-point
Discrimnation

Eyelid
Retractors
for Severe
Swelling

Circular Hooks
for Nasal
Foreign Body

Lid Everter
+ Elevator

FIGURE 3.7.   The multiple medical uses of paperclips.

■ **Fluoresceine:** Remove contact lenses first to avoid staining.
■ **Irrigation:** If don't have a Morgan lens, can use oxygen tubing hooked up to bag of LR.
■ **Seidel's Test:** For ruling out a ruptured globe. Paint the area of concern with thick fluorescein. If orange color is washed out to yellow by a waterfall of leaking fluid, the test is positive.

EARS, NOSE, AND THROAT

EARS

■ **Ear Foreign Body**
  - *Bead*: Curette, suction, dermabond on a cotton tip swab.
  - *Cotton*: Alligator forceps.
  - *Veggie*: No water; it may cause it to swell.
  - *Roach*: Warm 2% lidocaine or mineral oil followed by alligator forceps.

■ **Hematoma**: Aspirate with 18-gauge or IandD. Pack auricle with xeroform, then place a pressure dressing.

■ **Wax:** Irrigate with warm water using syringe and angiocath.

NOSE

■ **Nasal Foreign Body:** Snot rocket: Parent have child blow out while blowing into mouth and occluding other nare. Tools: speculum, curette, Fogarty, bent paperclip (see Figure 3.7).

■ **Anterior Epistaxis**
  - 0. Prepare gown, goggles, gloves, light, suction. Assess vitals.
  - 1. LET, Lido with epi or Afrin on cotton ball and local pressure with fingers or device x 15 min. If ineffective, at least it numbs for next part.
  - 2. Silver nitrate only works if bleeding has stopped and has risks, plus no proven benefit. Apply for only 5–10 seconds with rolling motion. Never use bilaterally. Alternate: Nose bleed QR: a powder salt that forms a crust (about $10).
  - 3. Packing: Antibiotic ointment on outside lubricates. Home on oral ABX. Leave in 2–3d. Alternates: FloSeal thrombin (about $180) or Thrombin-JMI (about $60).
  - 4. ENT: Call if previous doesn't work or if posterior bleed. Consider surgery or embolization.
  - 5. D/C: Prior to D/C, make sure patient can walk around ED and bend over without bleeding.
  - 6. If no packing, make sure to recommend Vaseline QID. NNT = 4 to prevent one revisit.

■ **Posterior Epistaxis:** Often post-operative. Can be very serious. Get ENT help early.
  - *Rx*: 14 Foley-tip cut + test, 4–8–20 ml air, gentle tension.
  - *Complications*: If posterior pack at risk for: hypoxia, ID, cardiac arrest.

■ **Septal Hematoma:** Call ENT. If none available, incise inferiorly and remove clot. Then pack nose.
  - *Anesthesia*: LET or cocaine. Aspirate with 20-gauge. If ineffective, IandD. Roll swab down septum to push blood out. Pack and start ABX. ENT f/u in 3–5d.

THROAT

■ **Abscess**
  - *Anesthesia*: Nebulized 2% lidocaine and/or hurricane or cetacaine spray.
  - *Preparation*: Suction with Yankauer.
  - *Good light*: Head lamp, laryngoscope, or lower half of lighted vaginal speculum.
  - *Avoid carotid*: Make needle guard: cut distal 1.5 cm off needle cap then replace it.
  - *Needle*: 18 gauge 3.5" spinal needle. Aim medially with bevel facing laterally.
  - *Location*: Try superior pole then if no pus, middle then inferior.
  - *Open more*: Blunt dissection into area of maximum fluctuance with a hemostat.
  - *Other*: Can use intracavitary ultrasound first to look for abscess in uncertain cases.

COMPARTMENT SYNDROME AND TENDONITIS

COMPARTMENT PRESSURE MEASUREMENT

■ **Sites:** Leg and forearm most common (see Table 3.5) > foot, thigh, gluteal > hand, abdomen, chest.

■ **Indications:** Suspicion for compartment syndrome.

■ **Contraindications:** Obvious compartment syndrome where measurement would cause delay to OR.

■ **Complications:** Infection, bleeding, tissue damage, false negative.

■ **Technique:** Patient fully supine or prone with compartment at heart level. Take 2–3 measurements. Muscles must be relaxed (may require sedation), 18 gauge needle perpendicular to skin—may need spinal needle for deep compartments. Confirm tip location by seeing rise in pressure during muscle contraction. Inject <0.3ml of sterile saline into compartment while measuring.

  ● *False high reading*: Needle tip in tendon, plugged catheter, faulty electronics.

  ● *False low reading*: Not in compartment, bubbles in lines, plugged catheter, faulty electronics.

■ **Devices:** Manometer can be made. Most centers should have at least one of the others below. May need to call OR if ED does not have own dedicated device.

  ● *Stryker*: Most accurate, most expensive. Set up, purge air w/ saline, zero device. Directions on back.

  ● *Manometer*: Mercury manometer is least expensive and easily put together but is least accurate.

  ● *Arterial line*: Arterial line system is better than a manometer.

  ● *Catheter*: Wick or slit catheter devices are rarely available.

■ **Timing:** Pressure peaks 6h after injury. Always measure serially if symptoms evolve. Muscle death in 4–12 h.

■ **Results**

  ● *< 10 mmHg*: Normal: Consult, use clinical judgement and repeat if status worsens.

  ● *10–30 mmHg*: Equivocal: consult, use clinical judgement and repeat if status worsens. Consider surgery for lower values if hypotensive or peripheral vascular disease.

  ● *> 30 mmHg*: Emergency surgery indicated.

TABLE 3.5. Muscle Compartments of the Forearm and Lower Leg

Compartment	Nerve	Motor	Sensory
Arm: Dorsal	Radial	Finger extensors	1st dorsal web space
Arm: Superficial volar	Ulnar	Superficial flexors	4th and 5th finger pad
Arm: Deep volar*	Median	Deep finger flexors	1st, 2nd, and 3rd finger pad
Leg: Deep posterior	Posterior tibial	Calf and toe flexors	Sole of foot
Leg: Superficial posterior**	None	Calf flexors	None
Leg: Anterior*	Deep peroneal	Foot dorsiflexors	1st dorsal web space
Leg: Lateral (peroneal)	Superficial peroneal	Foot eversion	Dorsal foot

* = Higher risk for compartment syndrome; ** = Lower risk for compartment syndrome

STEROID INJECTIONS FOR BURSITIS AND TENDONITIS

■ **Contraindications:** Infection, bleeding disorder. Avoid repeat injections. Prior injection in past 6 weeks.

■ **Medication:** Depot-Medrol: 5–15 mg for tendon sheath, 10–20 mg for medium bursa, 40–60 mg for large.

■ **Technique:** Call orthopedist first! There are complications. May add lidocaine. Z-track.

ARTHROCENTESIS AND JOINT INJECTIONS

GENERAL ARTHROCENTESIS

■ **Indications**
  - *Dx*: New onset effusion, arthritis, septic joint, occult fracture.
  - *Rx*: Remove hemarthrosis, instill medicine.

■ **Contraindications:** Relative: sepsis, coagulopathy (reverse first), prosthesis, overlying cellulitis (at least ABX first).

■ **Preparation:** Iodine then alcohol. Iodine must be dry to be more effective. Chlorhexidine likely better. Extensor side has fewer neurovascular structures. Traction to increase joint space.

■ **Tricks:** Use large butterfly needle or an angiocath, then remove needle.

ARTHROCENTESIS SITES

■ **Wrist:** 30° of flexion, traction, and ulnar deviation, 22-gauge dorsally just above meeting of extensor policis longus and 2nd digit extensor in the dimple. AVOID SNUFF BOX.

■ **Elbow:** 90° of flexion, pronation with palm on table. 22-gauge between lateral epicondyle and radial head. AVOID A MEDIAL APPROACH. Cause often gout, septic, pseudogout.

■ **Shoulder:** Hand in lap. 18–20 gauge. Anterior: inferio-lateral to coracoid. Alt. approach: lateral, posterior.

■ **Hip:** Ortho should do under fluoroscopy in OR.

■ **Knee:** 0° of flexion, relax quads. 18 gauge. Lift patella with thumb. Enter mid-patella or slightly superior of mid-patella medially (or laterally).

■ **Ankle:** Difficult. Keep foot plantar flexed. Use 20-gauge needle. Enter just medial to anterior tibial tendon in the medial malleolar sulcus. Must go in 2–3 cm.

■ **Toe/Finger:** 20° of flexion, traction. 22-gauge dorsally on side of central slip.

ARTHROCENTESIS RESULTS

■ **Cell Count:** Every reference has slightly different WBC numbers. The information in Table 3.6 is from Roberts and Hedges.
  - *RBCs*: DDx: Hemophilia, sickle cell, pseudogout, amyloid, RA, infection.
  - *WBC:* > 50,000 should Rx for septic even if crystals present (89% specific for septic joint), but 37% of septic joints have a WBC count less than 50,000 (only 63% sensitive).

TABLE 3.6.   Arthrocentesis Results by Condition

Condition	WBC Count	PMN %	Glucose (% serum)
Normal	< 200	< 25	> 95
OA/Trauma	< 4000	< 25	> 95
Crystal	2000–50,000	> 75	> 80
Inflammatory	2000–50,000	50–75	≈ 75
Septic	5000–50,000+	> 75	< 50
Prosthetic	> 1000	> 65	

Roberts JR, Hedges JR. *Clinical Procedures in Emergency Medicine.* 5th ed. Philadelphia: Saunders; 2009.

■ **Crystals:** Use a green top tube. Gout = negative needles; pseudogout = positive rhomboid. Crystals may be missed if lab doesn't look carefully and may dissolve with time.

METHYLENE BLUE INJECTION TO RULE OUT OPEN JOINT

■ **Indications:** Deep laceration near a joint. Contraindications: G6PD deficiency or obvious open joint.

■ **Technique:** Dilute 1 ml methylene blue in 500 ml sterile saline, inject—must use an 18 gauge needle. Look for extravasation (if present, Rx = IV ABX + formal wash-out in OR), aspirate extra
  - *Volume:* Until distended and uncomfortable: Guidelines: Knee: 30–50 ml; Elbow: 10–30 ml

DISLOCATIONS

DISLOCATIONS ABOVE THE WAIST

■ **General:** Position extremity to relax tendons. Good counter-traction is key. Always check neurovascular status before and after. Try local anesthesia before going to conscious sedation.

■ **Jaw**
  ● *Anterior:* Jaw stuck open, usually unilateral. Rx: Double glove. Patient seated, push down, and posterior. May need sedation.

■ **Finger**
  ● *Relocate*: Digital anesthetic block, wrist flexed if dorsal dlc, traction and gentle pressure.
  ● *Splinting*: DIP: 0–30°; PIP-dorsal: 15°; PIP-anterior: 50°; MCP-dorsal: 60°; MCP-anterior: 90°.

■ **Wrist**
  ● *Check:* Volar and median nerve OK?
  ● *Technique:* Finger traps > dorsiflex wrist and push in, then palmar flex.

■ **Elbow**
  ● *Posterior*: Palm to palm, clasp fingers and apply traction. Traction–countertraction with volar pressure distal. Splint elbow: 90–120°.

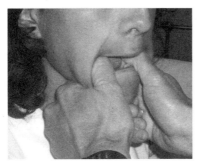
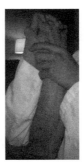

FIGURE 3.8. Mandible relocation: Wear gloves.   **FIGURE 3.9.** Elbow relocation.

  ● *Anterior*: Partial extension and traction. Splint elbow at 90–120°.
  ● *Nursemaids:* Hyperpronation method is less painful and better than flexion + supination

■ **Shoulder**
  ● *Lidocaine:* Use posterior approach to avoid deltoid nerve. Aim toward coracoid process. 20 ml 1% lidocaine with 20-gauge needle. Let sit for 10–20 min.
  ● *Anterior*: Cunningham: Interlock forearms, massage trapezius/deltoid, mild traction. Hennepin: Supine, external rotation, then over head, then down in front. Milch: External rotation to 90 + abduction to 90. Other: Traction–countertraction, Stimson, scapular manipulation. Splinting: Keep in 10 external rotation post reduction: Sling better than immobilizer.
  ● *Posterior*: Traction–countertraction, Stimson.
  ● *Inferior*: Traction–countertraction with slow arc to adduction, Stimson.

■ **Sterno-Clavicular Joint**
  ● *Anterior*: Towel under scapula, lateral arm traction, press on SC joint; figure-of-eight splint.
  ● *Posterior*: Towel roll, lateral arm traction, lidocaine, grasp with towel clamp.

DISLOCATIONS BELOW THE WAIST

■ **Hip**
- *General:* If out > 6 hr, risk of AVN much higher. Check sciatic nerve pre- and post-reduction. Tie patient's pelvis down to the bed with a sheet. Consider calling anesthesia. Post: CT pelvis for fx. Abduction pillow if admit, knee immobilizer if going home.
- *Posterior*
   1. Bed high, patient's butt at edge. Stand on floor with patient knee over MD's shoulder.
   2. Stimson: Patient prone hip on edge of bed. MD's knee on patient's calf.
   3. Patient on floor; slight external rotation; lift flexed knee.
   4. MD's foot on bed, MD's knee under patient's knee, use MD's calf to push up.
   5. MD's forewarm behind patient's knee, bend knee, pull, rotate hip in and out, lateral press.
- *Anterior:* Longitudinal traction and lateral force to thigh, then internal rotation.

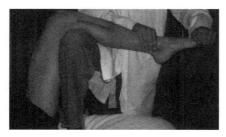

FIGURE 3.10.   Hip relocation.

■ **Knee**
- *Anterior:* Traction, lift femur anterior, avoid hyperextension; needs vascular study.
- *Posterior:* Longitudinal traction, lift tibia anterior, avoid hyperextension. Do vascular study.

■ **Patella**
- *Lateral:* Can use lidocaine intra-articular. Flex hip, extend knee, slow lateral pressure.

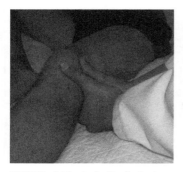

FIGURE 3.11.   Patella relocation: Have hips flexed.

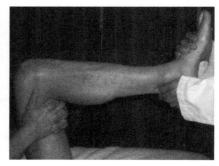

FIGURE 3.12.   Ankle relocation: Have knee bent.

■ **Ankle**
- *Posterior:* Knee bent to keep tendons lax. Plantar flex foot, apply traction, move anterior.
- *Anterior:* Knee bent to keep tendons lax. Dorsiflex foot, apply traction, move posterior.

FRACTURES AND SPLINTS

FRACTURE REDUCTION ANESTHESIA

Reduce stat if neurovascular compromise present.

- **Hematoma Block:** 10 cc 1% lido or 5 cc 2% lido; Contras: dirty skin, open Fx, children; Onset: 5–15 min; duration 1–2 hr +.
- **Beir Block:** IV lidocaine + pressure cuff to prevent systemic effect. Good but complex. Better anesthesia, but more risks for lidocaine toxicity.

SPLINTING

- **Duration:** 2–8 wks: cut tendon, fracture (joint above and below), open Fx: cover with betadine gauze; 6d: laceration, tendonitis, sprain; 4d: cellulitis, puncture/bite; 2d: abrasion/contusion.
- **Benefits:** Decreases pain, neurovascular injury and fat embolism.
- **Problems:** DVT, thermal burn, compartment syndrome, poor set, poor mold, stiffness.

TABLE 3.7.   Splinting

Splint	Indications	Layers	Coverage
Long arm post	Elbow, proximal forearm	8–10	MCP joint to proximal humerus
Volar	Wrist sprain, triquetral fx.	8–10	MCP joint to elbow
Sugar tong	Distal radius/ulna fx	8–10	MCP around elbow to MCP
Thumb spica	Scaphoid, lunate, thumb, 1st metacarpal	8–10	Thumb tip to mid forearm
Ulnar gutter	4th and 5th fingers or metacarpals	6–8	Beyond DIP to mid forearm
Radial gutter	2nd and 3rd fingers or metacarpals	6–8	Beyond DIP to mid forearm
Knee immobilizer	Knee derangement, hip relocation	N/A	High thigh to above ankle
Long leg	Knee Fx, tibia Fx, high ankle Fx	10–12	Buttock crease to ball of foot
Short leg	Most ankle Fx (not Maisonneuve)	10–12	Below knee to beyond toes
Cast shoe	Minor foot Fx, dancer's Fx, (not Jones fx)	N/A	Sole of foot

- **Padding:** Webril (two to four layers, more at bumps) and stockinet beyond and fold back. Pad edges. NO wrinkles.
- **Plaster:** Arms 8–10 layers; legs 12–15 layers. Laminate to increase strength. Exothermic reaction may cause burns: ↑risk: more layers, fast-set plaster, warmer water.
- **ACE:** Not too tight; can still get compartment syndrome with splint + ACE; tape both sides.
- **Mold:** Use palms, not fingers. Keep smooth. Do not move for at least 10 min.
- **Fingers:** Tips open to check circulation.

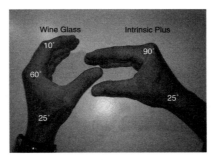

FIGURE 3.13.   Positions for splints.

LACERATIONS

GENERAL
Murmur: Gets ABX
- **Note:** "SAID EDS" (**S**terile, **A**nesthesia, **I**rrigate, **D**ebride, **E**xplore, **D**ress, **S**plint).
- **Warnings:** Misses: FB, nerve, tendon. Risk of infection if > 6h old (can use > 18h for face and head).
- **8-Hr Rule:** ↑Risk for infection: > 6 hr, ACEP clinical policy is 8–12 hr cutoff for primary closure.
- **Bites:** DEBRIDE. Cat: 1.5 cm incise > MD WASH IT; face or lip lac.: sew, ABX. Hand: don't sew.
- **Foreign Body:** Missed foreign body is the 5th leading cause of litigation for EPs. US good. CT will pick up wood in < 24 hr (> 48 hr wood absorbs water and can't be seen).

INFECTION
- **Rates:** All comers—3%; dog—5%; cat—15%.
- **Bites:** Don't sew primarily animal bite on hand, foot, leg, puncture.
- **Bugs:** Shoes: Pseudomonas. River/Lake: Aeoromonas. Sea: Vibrio. Wood: Enterobacter.
- **Prevention:** Debridement, irrigation, using tape or staples (loose closure doesn't decrease risk).
  - *Irrigation*: 7 psi if contaminated. Debride. Tap water = 45 psi and works fine. Don't do to puncture (spreads).
- **Increased Risk:** ESRD, ESLD, CHF; soak, epi, sutures, FB, edema, > 8 hr (but up to 18 hr may be OK if clean).
  - *Don'ts*: Don't soak, don't get any betadine in wound (cytotoxic).
- **Antibiotics:** +/–; "ABC's" (**A**ge > 8 hr, articular; **B**one; **C**rush, contam.), DM/PVD/Im, edema, foot, hand, hardware. Evidence+: GSW abdomen, open fracture, tendon, animal bite, murmur (ancef 2 g + gent), lymphedema. Consider: GSW extremity, dog bite, open tuft fracture, mouth/lip/gum, cartilage, >12–24h old.
- **Tetanus/dT:** Need if age > 14; DT or DPT age < 6.
  - *Contraindications*: F, neuro dx, prior rxn or pregnant (Tetanus alone usually OK).
  - *High risk*: > 8 hr, deep, burn, crush, puncture, ID, dirty, necrotic.
  - *Rx*: Unvaccinated: Tetanus immune globulin and dT now, dT again at 1 and 6 mon.

ANESTHETIC INJECTIONS
Intradermal more effective
- **Max. Doses:** Lidocaine 4.5 mg/kg (30 cc 1%), lido + epi 7 mg/kg (50 cc 1%), marcaine 2 mg/kg(70 cc 0.25%).
  - *Lido tox.*: Dizzy, tinnitus, tingle, nystagmus (Rx = O_2); seizure (Rx = benzo); shock (Rx = IVF, dopamine).
  - *Epinephrine tox.*: Vasospasm: Rx: phentolamine 0.5 ml (2.5 mg) + 0.5 ml of 1% lidocaine. Inject at same spot.
- **Benadryl:** Dilute 1:4; doesn't work well on face or palms. More painful to inject than lido. 5-min onset.
- **Bupivicaine:** Max: 2 mg/kg; lasts 4–8 hr. ACI: don't injure/burn skin. Contras: lip, digit-block (doesn't work).
- **Epinephrine:** NO: contaminated, infection risk, bad flap, vascular injury, (ears, toes, penis, nose, fingers).
- **Injecting:** Less pain with smaller needle, buffering, warming, slower injection, through wound edges.
- **Face:** Injection can distend tissues: nerve block after topical works well (mental nerve, etc.).
- **Fever:** Malignant hyperthermia: causes: succ., fluranes, curare, lidocaine, bupivicane, ketamine.

TOPICAL ANESTHETICS
Consider use of ice
- **LET/XAP:** Avoid: Eyes, > 4 cm lac. Onset coincident with skin blanch, usually 20' but 30'–1 hr better. Effectiveness: Face: 85%, extremities: 45%.
- **EMLA:** Onset 60 min; eutectic = lower melting point. Prilocaine can cause methemoglobinemia.
- **LMX-4:** Onset 30 min. Liposomal lidocaine 4% cream; 20% cheaper than EMLA.
- **Pain Ease:** Vapocoolant spray, lasts 60 sec, for IV access, vaccines, injections, 50¢/spray.
- **TAC:** Don't use on mucous membranes. LET preferred as safer, use.
- **Intra-Oral:** Lidocaine gauze held in place for 5–10 min or until numb.

REGIONAL ANESTHESIA: FACE

- ■ **Technique:** Elicit paresthesias then pull back slightly. Use 1–3 ml anesthetic.
- ■ **Cautions:** Remember nerves and vessels run together so always aspirate before injecting.
- ■ **Web:** www.nysora.com

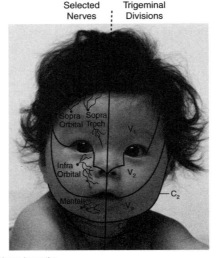

FIGURE 3.14.   Selected facial nerve innervation.
Source: © Photodisc and Pregerson, DB. *Quick Essentials Emergency Medicine 4.0.* ERPocketbooks.com; 2010:136.

■ Nerve Blocks

Suprorbital and Supratrochlear Nerves

- ● *Forehead*: Palpate notch medial to pupil.
- ● *Infraorbital nerve for upper lip*: Palpate divot even with pupil.
- ● *Mental nerve for lower lip*: Palpate divot even with pupil.
- ● *Inferior alveolar nerve for lower teeth*: In mouth opposite 1st and 2nd premolar.
- ● *Lingual nerve*: Base of tongue posterior and medial to most distal molar.
- ● *Intra-oral*: Lidocaine gauze held in place for 5–10 min or until numb.

REGIONAL ANESTHESIA: EXTREMITIES

Consider US guidance.

- ■ **Ultrasound:** Nerves look like grape cluster. Inject around nerve or into sheath but not into nerve.
- ■ **Transthecal:** Hand surgeons use frequently. Infusion of local anesthetic into flexor tendon sheath.
  - ● *Pros*: Away from nerves and vessels, single injection.
  - ● *Cons*: More pain, ↑damage if ID.
- ■ **Technique:** 5-ml syringe with 50% lidocaine/50% bupivicaine. Inject into palmar surface at proximal digital crease in midline. Insert to bone, then withdraw 2–3 mm and angle distally.
- ■ **Femoral:** Landmark is femoral artery 2 cm below inguinal ligament. Needle 45° cephalad, lateral to artery. Feel a "pop" from the fascia. Infiltrate 10–20 ml of bupivicaine: Onset 15'. Duration 3–8 hr.

POST-ANESTHESIA AND PRE-REPAIR

- **Cleaning:** Trim hair, debride, irrigate (H_2O_2 and alcohol very tissue toxic > 10% betadine (1% is maybe OK).
- **Hemostasis:** Arterial cuff: elevate arm > 1 min to exsanguinate, then inflate to SBP + 30, 2-hr max. duration. In wound: Figure 8, clamp and tie, cautery < 2 mm. Consider: tourniquet, surgicel, Monsel's, Drysol, Avatine, silver nitrate.
- **Explore:** NVI, tendons intact; "bottom of wound was visualized in a bloodless field through full range of motion and no foreign bodies or tendon injuries were seen." X-ray misses 40% 1/2 mm glass FB, so probe.

REPAIR GENERAL

Don't sew adipose

- **Exploration:** Palpate base, full range of motion in bloodless field, miss 40% 1/2 mm glass on X-ray so probe.
- **Hemostasis:** Artery: cuff: 2-hr max., SBP + 30; Figure 8, clamp and tie, cautery < 2 mm; running interlock.
- **Delayed 1°:** Clean and debride, then pack and dress. Keep closed 3–5d and clean and debride, then suture.
  - *Indication*: Infected, heavy soil contamination, bite, GSW, nonviable tissue.
- **Dermabond**
  - *Pros*: Faster, less painful, no return for removal, won't strangulate, keeps wound moist.
  - *Cons*: Tension, complex, crease > 10 cm, porphyria, bite, dirty, dense hair, deep, hands, mouth.
  - *Technique*: LET → clean → dry → open → apply four to five coats each larger than prior. Keep out of wound. Best edge apposition often obtained not by pushing edges, but by traction in-line with wound.
  - *Tricks*: Fold and cut hole in a Tagaderm to protect from dripping away. Aspirate into tuberculin syringe and apply with 24-gauge angiocath.
  - *ACI*: No ABX ointment. No swimming or sweating. 2d wound check. Will fall off in 7–10d.
  - *Complications*: Eyelid: ABX ointment to remove (water hardens it). Dehiscence: MUST do 2d wound check.
- **Staples:** Faster, less infection, more painful to remove. Linear lacerations. Avoid on hands and face.
- **Steri-strips:** Useful in small, low-tension wounds that might not even require closure at all. Useful to bolster wound edges in elderly patients. Useful to bolster wound edges in thin skin.
- **Suturing:** 3.0: scalp, sole, deep; 4.0: body, extremities; 5.0–6.0: face, neck. Subcuticular stitches may decrease keloid risk.
  - *Regular*: Prolene: better strength and tissue reactivity; Ethilon: better workability and knot security.
  - *Dissolving*: Mucosa: chromic gut: 7–10d. Buried: Vicryl. Others: Dexon, PDS. Peds: Use if doing conscious sedation to put in (esp. lip); face/lip: fast absorbing gut; skin: gut.
  - *Tension*: Vertical mattress, undermine, deep stitch.
  - *Eversion*: Best with horizontal mattress.
  - *Flap*: Modified horizontal mattress in tip. Elder: Steri-strip wound edge.
  - *Deep*: ↓Hematoma, dead space and tension; possibly better long-term cosmesis. Don't sew through adipose: ↑infection, no benefit.

TABLE 3.8.   Suture Type Comparison Table

Suture	Nylon	Prolene	Mersilene	Vicryl	Gut	Chromic Gut	Fast Gut
Filaments	mono	mono	multi	multi	mono	mono	mono
Absorbed in	N/A	N/A	N/A	60–90d	10–40d*	15–60d*	3–5d
Color	black	blue	white	white	tan	tan	tan
Uses	general	general	tendon	buried	peds	tongue	ped's face
Advantages	knot	strength	tendon	dissolves	dissolves	dissolves	dissolves

* Note: In mouth, plain gut absorbs in 3–5d and chromic gut in 7–10d.

SUTURE TALK

What you should talk about while suturing

■ **Inform:** Tell patient you are looking for tendon and nerve injuries and foreign bodies.

■ **Warn:** Small foreign bodies may be missed. Antibiotics don't prevent infection.

REPAIR OF HANDS AND FEET

■ **Dorsal:** Use horizontal mattress stitch to prevent wound inversion, which is common here. Extensor tendons are VERY superficial here. Assume injured until proven otherwise.

■ **Palmar:** Zone 2: PIP-palm; pad > nerve > artery > tendon; tendon runs with nerve.

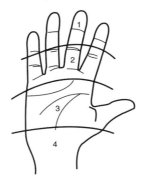

FIGURE 3.15.   Zones of the hand.

■ **History:** Position at injury: "Patient denies weakness, FB sensation, numbness, broken bone."

■ **Nerve:** Check 2PD. Rx: repair < 48 hr: 90% heal OK. No repair only 6% nerves grow back OK.

■ **Tendons:** Compare R&L, resistance test! Beware of a partial tendon laceration.

   ● *Extensor*: Tendon very superficial, usually cut. Pinky and thumb have duplicate tendons (easy to miss).

   ● *Rx*: Splint, call ortho to arrange to fix partial tendon lac > 50% in < 24–48 hr.

■ **Imaging:** Foreign body: XR is 90/90. May be visible on only one view. US: 40%/60%. CT: gold standard.

■ **Pitfalls:** No consult, no f/u hand 48 hr; misses: FB, partial tendon, 2nd FDS and EPL, buttonhole.

■ **Fingertip:** Replant proximal to DIP and all thumb/peds. Replants: 50% cold intolerance, skin fissures.

   ● *Viability*: If unsure about a partial avulsion, can debride. If it starts bleeding, it's probably viable.

■ **Nail Bed:** Don't need to remove unless nail bed is avulsed. Repair is difficult: use 6.0 absorbable.

   ● *Splint*: Use the removed nail x 3 wk: Maintains anatomy, covers sensitive area, maintains nail fold. Sew it in place at both lateral edges. Nail takes 4 mon. to regrow. Consider hand surgery for matrix graft; check for mallet finger carefully. Six months for nail to regrow; warn about possible permanent nail deformity.

■ **Punctures:** ID up to 15%, #1= staph; #1 osteo = pseudomonas.

   ● *Rx*: Nonweight bearing, Quinolone x 3d (no evidence so controversial), r/o FB is most imp

■ **Paint Guns:** Devastating injuries; infection, fibrosis, disability, and amputation all common. Digital block contraindicated. Need to go to OR stat.

■ **Ring Removal:** Should remove all rings on injured or infect hand as swelling could cut off circulation.

   ● *Trick*: Use soap or glass cleaner (this is what jewelers use) to slip it off. A ring cutter can also be used.

REPAIR OF FACE AND HEAD

■ **General:** Consider underlying anatomy: facial nerve, lacrimal duct, salivary duct. Mid face drains to CNS.

■ **Devil's Triangle:** Venous drainage of central face is toward brain. Infections here can cause CNS abscesses.

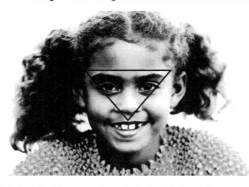

FIGURE 3.16.   Devil's triangle: Infections in this area have venous drainage directly toward the brain.
Source: © Photos.com

■ **Scalp:** Galea 4.0 nylon, muscle 4.0 vicryl; clip, don't shave hair.
- *Hair apposition technique (HAT):* Single twist of hair on both sides followed by tissue glue on hair. Contras: hair < 3 cm long, laceration > 10 cm, gross contamination, active bleeding, tension.

■ **Lip/Mouth:** Lac. < 1–2 cm usually heals well without stitches. Lido p 1st vermilion stitch; tooth FB in lip? Thru and thru: Check for tooth in lip. Close from inside to out.

■ **Tongue:** Often better to leave alone. Do sew lateral flaps. Difficult, consider stay suture or clip in tip. Lingual nerve block, tie stitches loosely because tongue swells. Use chromic gut.

■ **Eyelid:** Ophtho for: near eye (contractures), lid margin, duct, levator, fat shows (into orbit).

■ **Ear:** Prevent auricular hematoma; splint: wet cotton balls > gauze pack > head wrap; levaquin.

POST-REPAIR CARE

■ **Dressing:** Infection rates lower and healing faster when kept moist. Op-site better than gauze.
- *Peds:* Consider Steri-strip or Op-site to cover; prevents picking.
- *Pressure:* Pressure dressing x 48 hr for hematoma evacuation, scalp.
- *Tube gauze:* Improper/tight application can cause ischemia. Don't use more than two layers or pull or twist.

■ **Splinting:** Splint when possible tendon involvement or tension on wound near a joint.

■ **Recheck:** 48 hours is recommended timing for wound checks.

■ **Removal:** Timing: 5d: face; 15d: legs, joint; 10d: all others; don't rush it: tension, elderly, DM. Consider removing earlier, at 3–4d from face and placing Steri-strips.

INCISION & DRAINAGE, EXCISIONS

INCISION AND DRAINAGE

■ **General:** If > 2 cm ring of rubor = cellulitis; neck: call ENT, aneurysm?

■ **ABX 1st:** Septic, face, murmur/valve: amp 2 g + gent 30' before then amoxicillin 1.5g po 6 hr later.

■ **Confirm:** May do US or aspirate in equivocal cases. Aspiration may yield false negative.

■ **Anesthesia:** Analgesic if not driving, EMLA (especially for children), lidocaine injection.

■ **I&D:** Cut parallel to vessels and entire length of abscess unless cosmetic area. Break loculations.

   ● *Loop:* Two parallel incisions; tie loop with the packing and leave there for 7d. Good for selected abscesses; won't fall out and can bathe around it.

■ **Felon:** I&D on ulnar side of digits 2, 3, 4 or radial side of digits 1 or 5.

■ **Aftercare:** 24 hr f/u; 48 hr d/c packing; soaks; shower, splint, elevate (Q-tip and peroxide).

SUBUNGUAL HEMATOMA TREPHINATION

■ **Injury:** Often crush from hammer or door; very painful condition. Rule out fracture.

   ● *Types:* Simple: nail and margins intact; complex: with fracture, loss of tissue.

   ● *DDx:* If no trauma, consider: melanoma, nevus, splinter hemorrhage, Kaposi's sarcoma.

■ **Indications:** Trauma, painful, and nail edges intact; < 48 hr since injury or still severely painful.

■ **Contraindications:** Painless, nail to be removed for nailbed repair (size < 25% nail, > 48 hr since injury). Repair: Some recommend nailbed repair if > 50% involved; others only if nailbase is dislocated.

■ **Trephination:** Release of blood gives relief of pain; blood stays liquid for 36 hr +. OK, even if fracture.

   ● *Preparation:* Clean with betadine; finger block generally unnecessary. ABX optional even if fractured.

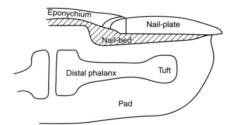

FIGURE 3.17.   Finger and nail bed cut-away.

   ● *Drill:* Essentially painless: use 18-gauge needle as a twist drill. Takes about 45 sec to do.

   ● *Melt:* May hurt; consider finger block; acrylic nails or alcohol prep may ignite; blood may clot in hole.

■ **Post:** Sterile dressing; nail may still be lost. Risk of nail deformity or infection higher if fractured.

INGROWN TOENAILS

■ **Preparation:** Digital block; soak for 20 min to soften nail. Sterile prep and drape.

■ **Complete:** Elevate nail from bed bluntly by inserting closed iris scissors and spreading or using a shim. Make sure to adequately dissect proximal corner(s). Splint nail fold open for 1 wk with petroleum gauze.

■ **Partial:** Remove involved two-fifths of nail.

■ **Alternatives:** Warm soaks and distal corner elevation.

■ **Prevention:** Cut nails straight across. Avoid tight shoes.

PROCEDURAL SEDATION BASICS

PRESEDATION CONSIDERATIONS

- ■ **Note:** Always adequately treat pain before titrating the sedation agent.
- ■ **Contraindications**
  - ● *Absolute:* Respiratory distress, unstable vitals, AMS, questionable airway, ASA class 5.
  - ● *Relative:* < 6 months, old, obese, pregnant, drugs, EtOH, sleep apnea, COPD, heart. ASA class 3 or 4, comorbidities, disease, prior anesthetic troubles, difficult airway.
- ■ **Pediatrics:** Have appropriate sized airway equipment at bedside. Double-check dosing. *Higher risk:* less pulmonary reserve, depth of sedation harder to assess.
- ■ **NPO Status:** For emergent procedures, no data to support that fasting decreases complications. ASA recommendations for elective procedures: *Solids:* 6–8 hr; *Liquids:* 4 hr; *Clears:* 2 hr.
- ■ **Airway Classes:** 1. See tip of uvula; 2. See sides of uvula; 3. See top of uvula; 4. See none of uvula. *Neck:* Check sniffing position and thyromental space: If < three finger breadths may be difficult.
- ■ **Set-Up Check:** IV/SAT/CM/BP; RT PRESENT: suction, airway, BVM, code cart. Drugs: atropine, flumazenil, narcan, $ETCO_2$ monitors

TABLE 3.9.   Pre-Sedation Considerations

ASA Class	Examples	Recommendation
1. Normal, healthy patient	No systemic disease	Procedural sedation OK
2. Mild systemic disease	Mild HTN, mild DM, sinusitis	Procedural sedation OK
3. Severe disease	Bad DM or HTN, RI, CAD, CVA	Anesthesiology consult
4. Incapacitating/life threat	ESRD, bad COPD, class 3 CHF	Anesthesiology or OR
5. Moribund	Not expected to survive 24 hr	Go to OR

IN-PROCEDURE CONSIDERATIONS

- ■ **Moderate:** Patient can be aroused by loud noise. Airway protection and ventilatory function not impaired.
- ■ **Deep:** Patient not aroused by noise. Airway protection and ventilatory function may be impaired.
- ■ **Assistance:** Must have trained and certified individual other than primary MD to monitor patient.
- ■ **Monitoring:** Vitals, monitor, O_2 sat. and alertness q 5 min for 30 min p last dose then q 15 x 30 min.
- ■ **Dosing:** Start with analgesic and titrate to effect; then add sedative and titrate to effect. Give agents slowly. ↓Dose in: "CLOCK" (**C**NS, **L**iver, **O**ld, **C**ardiac, **K**idney)
- ■ **Complications:** Resp: Hypoxia, hypercarbia, stridor, laryngospasm, apnea, CNS injury, death; Other: emesis, low BP or HR, aspiration, agitation, emergence reaction, abdo pain, HA.
- ■ **Corrections:** Resp: Stimulate patient, reposition airway, bag ventilation >> intubation; Other: antiemetics, rescue position, observation, IV fluids.
- ■ **Reversal:** Titrate reversal agents carefully to prevent side effects. If used must monitor an extra 2 hr.
- ■ **Death Causes:** Dosing error, multiple or long-acting agents, inadequate observation.

POST-PROCEDURE CONSIDERATIONS

- ■ **Desaturation:** Patient most likely to desaturate after the procedure when the painful stimulus is gone.
- ■ **Discharge:** Must monitor at least 30 min after last IV dose or 90 min after last IM dose.
  - ● *Criteria:* Vitals, O_2 sat., orientation, ability to follow commands, swallow, gag. Able to walk. All these must be stable and normal or at baseline. No driving for 24 hr.
- ■ **Documenting:** Review of H&P, consent, preprocedure assessment form, NPO status, ASA class, doses, complications, post-procedure, monitoring, physician intraservice time.

SECTION 4 ■ DIAGNOSES, DISPOSITIONS, AND LAWS

DIAGNOSES AND PITFALLS

MAKING A DIAGNOSIS
- **Spectrum:** In the ED, always assume the worst until proven otherwise.
- **Parsimony:** The simplest explanation is most likely to be true.
- **Billing:** List the most serious diagnosis first. Mention if acute, chronic, or acute on chronic. Avoid "normal exam," "medical screening exam," or "med refill" as they are nonbillable. OK to use a symptom or the chronic disease they need the refill for.

DIAGNOSTIC ERRORS AND SOME CAUSES
- **Anchoring:** Locking onto certain features of presentation early and failing to adjust to new info
- **Availability Bias:** Tendency to diagnose conditions that most easily come to mind
- **Communication:** Poor communication is the No. 1 cause of error in the ED. Collaboration helps.
- **Confirmation Bias:** Tendency to search for and/or interpret new data in way that confirms prior opinion.
- **Diagnostic Inertia:** Taking the diagnosis given by a prior physician as fact.
- **End-of-Shift Bias:** Short-cutting workup toward end of shift in order to finish and go home.
- **Framing:** Boxing in your thinking in a way that prevents thinking outside the box.
- **Ignoring Red Flags:** Not addressing all abnormal findings or test results. If it doesn't fit, try to explain.
- **Incomplete History:** Cutting corners on history taking due to time constraints, etc.
- **Labeling:** Not taking complaint seriously because patient labeled "frequent flyer," "drug seeker," etc.
- **Ockham's Oversight:** Often there is more than one disease process culminating in the patient's condition.
- **Overconfidence:** Believing you know more than you do; acting on hunch/opinion rather than fact
- **Premature Closure:** Making a diagnosis prior to analyzing or reconciling all of the data
- **Red Herring:** A fact or finding that leads you astray and off the scent of the culprit condition
- **Search Satisfied:** Calling off the search once something found, thus missing second insult or disease.
- **Smoking Gun:** Most immediately apparent cause of the problem
- **Triage Bias:** Letting the nurse's opinion influence or prejudice your own evaluation
- **Uncertainty:** If you are unsure about the patient, get a consult.

THE "TEN COMMANDMENTS" OF EMERGENCY MEDICINE
1. Secure the ABC's first
2. In an altered patient use glucose and narcan
3. Assume the worst until proven otherwise
4. Don't send an unstable patient to X-ray or CT
5. Address all red flags
6. Be the patient's advocate
7. Read nurses' notes and listen to their concerns
8. Trust no one, double check everything
9. Don't cut corners at the end of your shift
10. If you're not sure, double check or look it up

ED TOP MISSES AND COMMON REASONS

- **Fractures**: 19%, no X-ray done, subtle fracture, 2nd fracture not noticed
- **Infections**: 15%, CXR negative pneumonia (up to ¼), no LP done, bacteruria without pyuria
- **MI/ACS**: 10%, atypical presentation, painless, normal EKG, normal troponin
- **Cancer**: 9%, no f/u arranged for pulmonary nodules, minor GI bleed, etc.
- **Stroke**: 8%, atypical (esp. thalamic), chameleon, posterior circulation, CT negative, TIA
- **PE**: 5%, painless (large PEs), normal vital signs (small PEs), no risk factor, CT miss rate = 17%
- **Appendicitis**: 5%, atypical, poor return instructions, sent home on narcotics, retrocecal
- **Other Misses**: Perforated ulcer, epidural abscess, PTX, AAA delay in care, iritis, knee dislocation, CO poisoning, aortic dissection, carotid dissection, vertebral dissection, UTI, delayed subdural from coumadin, Fitz-Hugh-Curtis, early cholecystitis; peripheral vascular disease, testicular torsion

TABLE 4.1.   Some High-Risk Symptoms and Examples of Standard of Care

Symptoms	High Risk Disease	Standard of Care
Abdo Pain	Appy	Serial exams
Flank Pain	AAA	Be fast in case AAA
Testicle	Torsion	Don't delay. Urology consult
Wound	Tendon laceration, FB	Check carefully, and if unsure f/u with specialist
Crush	Compartment syndrome	Ortho to ED
Headache	SAH	Doing the LP

BOUNCEBACK RISKS

Rate < 72 hr is about 3%

- **Abnormal D/C Vitals**: Especially tachycardia or low BP
- **Flare of Chronic Dz**: CHF, COPD, CNS
- **Barriers to Return**: Resources, lives far away, substance abuse, mental disease
- **Atypical Sx**: Painless, early in process, subtle findings, extremities of age

DISPOSITION-HOME

■ Patient Condition

Do not use the word "stable."

- *Good*: Vitals OK, normal LOC, comfortable
- *Serious*: Vitals deranged or unstable, patient ill
- *Fair*: Vitals OK, normal LOC (uncomfortable)
- *Critical*: Vitals bad, patient may be altered, poor Px
- *NOTE*: If discharging home, for the most part use "Good" as the condition.

■ Home and After-Care Instructions (ACI)

- *Reality*: Patients may understand or remember only a fraction of what you tell them.
- *Document*: Counseled on Dx or lack thereof, Rx, need for f/u, possible complications, reasons to return. If patient requesting to go. All questions answered, if d/w PMD: "Case reviewed with nurse at dispo."
- *Checklist*: Lives alone? VS? Walks, PO trial, pain gone, distance, car, phone, F/U, family. If unsure: Have PMD come in or wait until 9 AM to talk to PMD. Get a consult.
- *Family*: Make sure family members with patient are comfortable with plan. Address all concerns.
- *Analgesia*: Give 3 days narcotics max. Best to avoid sending home with narcotics if diagnosis uncertain.
- *Cards*: Consider giving the patient a card with your number or e-mail if they have further questions.
- *ACI*: "FARMS" (**F**/U [time specific], **A**CI forms, **R**eturn to ED conditions. **M**eds, **S**pecial). Use colored paper. Keep duplicate on chart. Best if MD gives ACI and signs. Best to have friend or family member present for exit interview.
- *Patient want*: Exit interview with MD, to know Dx, test results, what to watch for, specific f/u, printouts.
- *Simplify*: No abbreviations, or medical jargon; 6th-grade level. 50% of lawsuits related to poor ACI.
- *F/U*: ALWAYS recommend f/u with SPECIFIC time frame. Last MD to see patient liable for a missed condition. "Return immediately if worse or . . . . See your doctor in the morning."
- *Wound*: Warn patient about possible missed: FB, Fx, partial tendon injury

■ Workers' Compensation Discharges

- *Company*: Check the company profile for special instructions, such as drug testing. If not found, ask.
- *History*: Mechanism, cause, onset, workplace conditions and demands, nonwork-related factors
- *Cause*: Give your opinion if more likely than not a work-related cause.
- *First aid*: Less work for all as nonreportable to OSHA. Employer must make the call, but if prescriptions strength meds used to treat, cannot qualify.
- *Work status*: Duration should be by calendar day, without consideration for holidays. Avoid "off work." Instead recommend limitations and employer is responsible from there.
- *Referrals*: Not to private MD (though can call for advice). Employer responsible for appropriate referral if nonemergent.
- *Treatment*: Can order physical or occupational therapy or worksite ergonomic evaluation.

WORKERS' COMP DICTATION*: MD'S 1ST REPORT, CALIFORNIA

17. Patient description of events
18. Subjective complaints
19. Objective: Exam and tests
20. Diagnosis. Toxins: Y/N
21. Findings consistent with Hx: Y/N**

22. Delay in recovery: Y**/N
23. Treatment rendered
24. Further Rx required: Y**/N
25. Admission? If so, location?
26. Work: Off/Modified/Regular

* Patients with work-comp and nonwork-comp issues need two charts.

** Please explain and give dates where applicable.

DISPOSITION HOME: AMA, REFUSALS, AND DECISION-MAKING CAPACITY

Against medical advice (AMA) is a type of informed refusal.

■ **5 Steps**
- 1. Must be of adult years and sound mind (no slurring, confusion, hypotension)
- 2. Must explain risks, benefits, and alternatives in language they can understand.
- 3. Always involve family, friends, and/or PMD and document it; may help to convince.
- 4. Document patient's reason for refusal and solutions offered.
- 5. Get signatures of patient and family. If won't sign, document why.

■ **Solutions**
- If pets locked at home, get the Humane Society to go to house to get them.
- If someone needs to pick up children, call police to do it.
- Rarely need psychiatry input, but may help if depression/psychosis is affecting decision.
- Negotiate a compromise if possible. Always give appropriate Rx, ACI, and f/u even if AMA.
- Part as friends. Make sure they know they can return.

■ **Document**
- "Warned"; "seriousness and urgency explained"
- DON'T LIST RISKS but may write "discussed risks with emphasis on . . ."

■ **Myths**: That insurance won't cover an AMA discharge

■ **Capacity**: Competence is a legal term decided by the court. "Decision-making capacity" better. Can be partial or depend on complexity of decision; can change, psych hold doesn't negate
- *Factors*: Cognition, judgment, understanding, ability to choose and explain reasons, stability of choice. Understand and explain risks/benefits or alternatives or no treatment.
- *Mini-Mental Status Exam (MMSE)*: Score < 19: Likely incompetent; Score > 25: Likely competent.
- *Worry if*: Age < 18, psychotic, developmental delay (intoxication), reasoning based on irrelevant info. Can't paraphrase, unclear thinking/speech, nursing notes incriminating, MMSE < 19, low BP
- *Psych Dz*: Does not usually affect capacity. Schizophrenic may understand issues at hand. Be careful if a suicidal patient refuses care.
- *Help*: Though not necessary, ethics committee may be helpful, as may risk management.
- *Solutions*: If decision can wait, treat any reversible medical or psychiatric disease contributing to AMS. Involve family: spouse > adult children > parents > siblings > other relatives
- *Intoxicated*: Restrain and document "confused" until released. Then document "medically safe to d/c."
- *Document*: "Not lucid, appears confused, confused per family." Document actions.

■ **Negotiation**: Involve the family, PMD, clergy, etc. Find the best Plan B you can. Try to let the patient know you are on their side; try not to argue with them but to help them.

■ **Surrogates**: If patient refuses and lacks capacity, must look for surrogate decision maker or proxy. An advanced directive or surrogate decision maker has priority in directing medical decisions.

■ **Trust**: Establishing trust through good communication may prevent or change refusals. Pay attention and listen to the patient. Show empathy.

ELOPEMENT

■ **Reason**: Document suspected reason if known.

■ **Search**: Search required: waiting room, bathrooms, smoking area. Document search and security called. If patient not located, call contact phone number and document it.

■ **Police**: Call police if intoxicated patient elopes or if opiate OD elopes within 2h of receiving Narcan.

ANALGESIA AND DRIVING

■ Analgesics

- *Abuse*: Analgesics > tranquilizers > stimulants > sedatives
- *Catch-22*: You can be held negligent and/or sued for oligo-analgesia, but the "model policy" emphasizes MDs have a responsibility to minimize narcotic abuse.
- *Document*: Poor records are a key factor in disciplinary measures for narcotic issues.
- *Drug seeker*: Forgery, sells drugs, alcohol abuse, noncompliance, dose escalation, multiple physicians. Deterioration in function at work or at home, reluctance to have tests or referrals, won't give PMD's name, visiting town and forgot meds, lost prescription, meds stolen, in a rush, etc. Sx: Complaints: kidney stone, headache, toothache, or back pain. Tricks: Photocopy their ID, check to see if their phone number is real. Insist to talk to their ride home.
- *Tips*: Can refuse to Rx narcotics if legitimate concern about misuse, but must refer to specialist. You can be sued for inadequate treatment of pain. Legitimate patients agree to you contacting their doctor or pharmacy and will provide their ID. Diverters tend to avoid, refuse, or become angry with these requests.
- *NSAIDs*: Proven for gout and rheumatoid conditions, renal/biliary colic, menstrual cramps. Risks: GI bleed, renal, MI, slowed healing in bones (? sprains), mild blood thinning

■ Impaired Driving and DMV Notification

- *Don't drive*: Sedatives, antihistamines, narcotics, eye patch, eye disease, syncope, vertigo. Document: "Patient told not to drive and has a ride home."
- *Notify DMV*: Any condition that could cause a lapse of consciousness or altered mental status. Conditions: Sz, syncope, dementia, DM, dysrhythmia, CNS tumor, narcolepsy, sleep apnea, medications; TIA, near syncope, hypoglycemia, vertigo, neuro disease, MS, psychiatric, family concerns. Consider: Bad arthritis, visual conditions. If drunk, call police.

TABLE 4.2.   Analgesic Comparison Table

Opiates	Ob/l	Equiv. Dose* End	Peak	Contras and (Cautions)	Side Effects and (Notes)
Darvocet❹	c/?	2 tabs	4–6 hr	(RI, L, Coum, CBZ)	OD danger: sz, dysr, death
Demerol❷	+/?	70 mg	3–5 hr	MAOI (Libby Zion), BHT	Sleep, dizzy, RR, BP, retention
Dilaudid❷+	c/?	1 mg	4–5 hr; 20 min	(Peaks at 20')	BM (NO HM release)
Lorcet❸	+/-	5 mg (1 tab)	4–5 hr	(See opiates and Tylenol)	(See opiates and Tylenol)
Lortab❸	+/-	5 mg (1 tab)	4–5 hr	(See opiates and Tylenol)	(See opiates and Tylenol)
methadone❷	c/?	7 mg	12–24 hr	(Rifampin lowers level)	↑QT, (Addict: 20–120 mg qd)
morphine❷	c/?	7 mg	4–5 hr; 40min	↑ICP, MAOI, (peaks at 40')	RR, BP, constip, V, sed
Oxycodone❷	c/?	5 mg (1 tab)	4–5 hr	hypopnea	constipation, sedation, N, V
Vicodin❸	+/?	5 mg (1 tab)	4–5 hr	↑ICP, (RI, L, thyroid, crine)	BM, delirium, retention
Vicoprofen❸	-/?	5 mg	4–5 hr	↑ICP, (RI, L, thyroid, crine)	Hydrocodone 7.5+ Ibu 200

* Equivalent doses: 1 tab Vicodin = 1 mg Dilaudid IV = 7 mg morphine IV = 75 mcgs Fentanyl IV.
❷: DEA Schedule 2 Drug, ❸: DEA Schedule 3 Drug, ❹: DEA Schedule 4 Drug
Source: Pregerson DB. *A to Z Pocket Pharmacopoeia.* ERPocketbooks.com: 58.

ADMISSIONS

■ Admission Decisions and Bed Type

- *Document*: "The case was discussed in detail with admitting MD, including need for...."
- *Lower threshold*: Unsure Dx, severe, unreliable patient, reduced immunity, pregnant, emesis, DM, VS bad; lives far from care, lives alone, psychiatric disease, tempo of disease, prior outcomes
- *Conflicts*: If disagree with PMD, get a consultant as a tie breaker or go up the chain of command.
- *ICU*: BP < 90, HR > 120, unstable, status epilepticus; unable to use call button; unable to protect airway if vomit. Systems: CNS, CV (get troponin), resp., endocrine, F/E/N, GI, heme, ID. Prevention: "HIPS" (**H**$_2$ blocker, **H**eparin, **H**ead of bed, **I**V/lines, **P**ressure sores, leg **S**queezers)
- *Telemetry*: Defibrillator firing, 2° and 3° AV block, long QT, ACS, r/o MI, dysr, CHF flare, syncope; severe electrolyte abnormalities, abnl ABG, frequent VS, CVA (all), OD, early sepsis; GI bleed, massive transfusion (↓Ca, ↑K)
- *Med/Surg*: OK for: low-risk CP with nl EKG, stable PE, asthma, mild infections, minor transfusion
- *Observation*: < 24 hour admit needed. Encouraged by Medicare and Medicaid. Can be 8–24–(48)h. Examples: Chest pain, CHF, asthma, syncope, head injury, abdo pain, back pain, TIA, altered, F, AGE. Caveats: If you admit as observation, you might still have an EMTALA risk. If you don't use observation and should have, payment might be affected.

■ Physician Quality Reporting Initiative (PQRI) or Core Measures

- *Pneumonia*
  Cognition: Mental status
  Vital Signs: O$_2$ sat. and vitals
  Vaccines: Pneumovax and flu: screen or give
  Cultures: Blood cultures prior to antibiotics
  Smoking: Cessation counseling
  Antibiotics: Appropriate ABX < 4 hr from triage time
- *Acute Myocardial Infarction*
  Aspirin: At arrival and prescribed at discharge
  Beta Blocker: Retired
  ACEI: For LV systolic dysfunction
  Time: Thrombolytics < 60 min, PTCA < 90 min
  Smoking: Cessation counseling
- *Syncope*
  EKG: EKG for all syncope patient
- *Stroke*
  TPA: tPA considered for all CVA < 4.5 hr

- *Congestive Heart Failure*
  Echo: LV functional assessment
  ACEI: For LV systolic dysfunction
  Smoking: Cessation counseling
  ACI: Discharge instructions including six specific recommendations
- *Pediatric Asthma*
  Beta Agonists
  Steroids
  Home plan
- *Central Lines*
  Sterility: Cap, mask, gown, gloves, barriers
  Chlorhexidine skin prep
- *ICU Prevention*
  Pneumonia: Elevate head of bed
  Peptic Ulcer: Medical prophylaxis
  DVT: Prophylaxis

■ Admission Holding Orders

- *Recommended*: EPs NOT write holding orders
- *Mnemonic*: "ADC VAN DIMPL"
  Admit: Observation, med/surg, telemetry, ICU
  Diagnosis: No abbreviations
  Condition: Good, fair, poor, serious, critical
  Vitals: How often, neuro checks, pulse ox, monitor, daily weights
  Activity: Bed rest, bathroom with assist, ad lib
  Nursing: What to call MD for (vitals, etc.)
  Diet: NPO, cardiac, ADA with calories, renal, soft
  IV: IV fluid orders
  Meds: PRNs, standards, consider holding certain meds (i.e., metformin if getting a CT)
  Prophylax: Heparin? H$_2$ blocker? laxative?
  Labs: Based on admitting Dx

INFORMED REFUSALS FOR ADMITTED PATIENTS

See Disposition Home: AMA, Refusals, and Decision-Making Capacity and Elopement sections on page 104.

■ **Indications**: Patient refusing test, procedure, treatment, referral, admission to hospital, etc.

■ **Document**: There are specific forms for this. In a pinch consider making your own or using an AMA form (even if patient is admitted)

■ **Five Steps**
- 1. Must be of adult years and sound mind (no slurring, confusion, hypotension...).
- 2. Must explain risks, benefits, and alternatives in language they can understand.
- 3. Always involve family, friends and/or PMD and document it. May help to convince.
- 4. Document patient's reason for refusal and solutions offered.
- 5. Get signatures of patient and family. If won't sign, document why.

■ **Battery**: Unconsented touching. Do not commit battery. If the patient is not lucid, however, you may use implied consent.

■ **Religious Reasons**: May transfuse against will in some states if AMS, incompetent, pregnant, or has a dependent

INVOLUNTARY ADMISSIONS

■ **Psychiatric Holds**

Some of these laws are state/county specific.

- *Voluntary:* Less coercive, aids therapeutic alliance, ups patient involvement and buy-in, respects autonomy
- *72-hour hold*: Known as a 5150 in California. Immediate danger to self or to others or gravely disabled from a psych dz. Medical: Not used for medical treatment; may still be competent to make MEDICAL decisions. Agents: Can be placed by psych attending, peace officer, crisis team, "other designee" of county. GD: Gravely disabled: unable to provide food, clothing, or shelter and won't allow others to do for them; untreated medical problems do not count; must be caused by psychiatric dz. Drunk: In some cases, patient must no longer be under influence of drugs for 72-hr hold to be assessed. Minors: Parent may not prevent a valid hold.
- *Tarasoff*: If patient states intention to kill a specific person, you must notify police AND that person
- *D/C hold*: Only a psychiatrist who does a face-to-face evaluation can discontinue a hold.

■ **Restraints**

- *Indication*: Necessary for patient or provider safety and alternate methods not sufficient. Intoxicated patient or heroin OD < 2 h after Narcan tries to elope. Med-Surg: Patient trying to pull out lines, demented, fall risk trying to get out of bed. Good for 24 h. Behavioral: Combative, need for hard restraints. Good for 4h if age > 18, 2h if age 9–17 y, 1h if age < 9y
- *Document*: Need, reason, alternates tried
- *Ordering*: MD must complete written order within 1 hr of application
- *Application*: Nurse or MD; security officers should not apply or remove restraints. Consider patient privacy, dignity, and respect. Use the least-restrictive restraint that will work.
- *Assessment*: Behavioral restraints require q15 min patient assessment and continuous monitoring
- *Renewal*: Med-Surg: q24h; behavioral: age > 18: q4h, age 9–17: q2h, age < 9: q1h; remove restraints as soon as is safe
- *Injuries*: All need to be documented and reported.
- *Chemical*: Cannot be used without consent unless an emergent reason is documented; must first attempt to use less-restrictive interventions (document it)
- *Alternates*: Freedom splints, which are like knee immobilizers on the elbow, are not considered restraints. Immobilization for an exam; treatment or procedure does not constitute restraints. Police use of handcuffs is their responsibility.

■ **Child Protective Services (CPS) and Department of Health Services (DHS)**

- *CPS*: If parents refusing necessary care, call CPS immediately to inquire about holding child. Call police as well. "I'll see my doctor tomorrow" may be a lie.
- *DHS*: Patient with TB or other public health risk can be admitted involuntarily if necessary. Need DHS to request; calling protects you; not calling = big liability

TRANSFERS OUT AND THE HOMELESS

■ **CMS**: Center for Medicare + Medicaid Services.

■ **CoP**: Medicare Conditions of Participation

■ **EMTALA**: Emergency Medical Treatment and Labor Act.

  ● *Violations*: Untreated severe pain, no screening exam, even if waiting in ED for PMD

  ● *Illegal transfer/discharge*: Cases that are referred to specialist, then turned away at the office; can subpoena peer-review materials for EMTALA case

■ **Definitions**: "Come to the hospital" = within 250 yards of campus. Medical Screening Exam (MSE): Offer to everyone and document if refused (even if just the pelvic); must be the same as for your best paying patients. In ED, emergency condition presumed until proven otherwise, even if just a med refill request.

■ **Transfers:** To another hospital, to an office, or to home can all be considered as transfers by EMTALA.

  ● *Mode*: Private auto NEVER appropriate. Only use if you have a written refusal to go by ambulance.

  ● *Stability*: Stabilize as much as you can first. If transferring by ACLS for safety, then NOT stable. OK: Continuity of care, higher level of care, patient request Cons: Average of a 5-hr delay in care To Office: "Discharge and go to..." are generally considered improper EMTALA transfers. DO NOT TREAT THIS AS A DISCHARGE. This is actually a transfer for specialized care. Complete transfer forms, document why (higher level of care). "Return if not seen." If they do not need to be seen the same day, discharge more likely to be OK. Don't: Uterine contractions, patient need OR, untreated pain, for MD convenience, unstable psych, angina, CP, appy/SBO if any red flag (peds, 2nd visit, pain > 24 hr, fever, rebound) Document: Stable, risks/benefits/alts., accepting MD, on call MD who didn't respond, vital signs

■ **Call Panel:** DO NOT discuss insurance status. The panel physician should know this is not appropriate 30 min to respond, document name if no show. On-call must find replacement if unavailable. EP, not admitting MD or consultant, decides if consultant must come to ED, not debatable. Delay if in surgery is defensible, but starting elective cases or finishing office patients isn't.

■ **Office F/U:** Usually a bad idea. On-call must come in if requested. If refusal, use chain of command. Patient shouldn't go to office unless it's on-campus or has special facilities not available to ED. EMTALA does not apply to office setting. If patient denied care, you will likely be cited. If hospital bylaws require on-call to render f/u visit, EMTALA will enforce it. Patient must be accompanied by staff if going to an on-campus office. If forced to transfer an unstable patient, explain why and name consultant who refused to come in.

■ **Admitted:** Once admit order placed, EMTALA doesn't usually apply, unless admitted to avoid EMTALA.

■ **Homeless Patients and EMTALA:** If homelessness documented, so must be all the following.

  ● *Consent*: Signed patient consent

  ● *Follow-up*: Like all patients, must receive a discharge plan including f/u care

  ● *Clothing*: Must provide clothing and shoes

  ● *Medicine*: It is recommended that you provide a 30d supply of meds if patient cannot afford.

  ● *Transport*: Don't send across county lines. Taxi not recommended (won't wait to see if patient got into shelter)

  ● *Other*: Psychiatric and social work evaluations and/or referrals

  ● *John Doe*: Make sure they are not a missing person. Get social work, police, and/or psych involved.

TRANSFERS IN

■ **Accepting Higher Level of Care Transfers**

  ● *Basics*: You must comply with EMTALA; must have capacity to treat to accept

  ● *Conditions*: No conditions may be placed on acceptance, especially financial ones. However, suggestions in the interest of patient safety OK.

  ● *From*: Transfer may come from anywhere in the continental U.S.; even if patient is in-patient at outside hospital, duty to accept likely still applies

  ● *To*: Patients may come to ED or be a direct admit. If direct admit, admitting physician must be physically present when patient arrives.

  ● *Exceptions*: Accept unless unable to provide necessary care or ER on diversion can't direct admit. KNOW YOUR LOCAL HOSPITAL POLICIES ON THIS. Get help from your director or charge nurse if unsure.

■ **Accepting Lateral Transfers**

  ● *Basics*: Lateral transfers are usually processed identically to a direct admission from the community. They go through the admitting department or house supervisor after hours.

HAND-OFFS AND TRANSITIONS IN CARE

■ **Pass-ons**: By definition involve a gap in continuity of care and are common causes of medical errors; not well studied, JCH getting involved. NEVER leave before relief arrives; this is patient abandonment. Could lose your license.

■ **Benefits**: Team-building function, chance for 2nd-opinion with fresh eyes.

■ **Pitfalls**: Inadequate communication causing errors; lack of "ownership" of patient by 2nd MD

■ **Solutions**: Standardization of pass-ons, face to face, two-way communication, chance for questions. SBAR: method for handoff: situation, background, assessment, recommendation. Visit bedside and introduce patient to new MD, esp. if the dispo. is still undecided. Don't rush it, verbal AND written exchange, use of standardized forms or computer program. Involve nurses, minimize distractions, checklist for tasks, keep an open mind to suggestions. Read back to verify communication. Have oncoming MD sign chart to promote "ownership."

■ **Nursing**: Clarify which orders are completed and which are pending.

DEATH, DNR, AND PALLIATIVE CARE

■ **Declaring Brain Death**
  - *Step 1*: R/O reversible causes: sedatives, paralytics, hypothermia, metabolic, hypotension, hypoxia
  - *Step 2*: R/O cortical activity and brainstem reflexes: painful stimuli, light, corneal, gag, B calorics; apnea test: give 100% O_2 then off vent and ABG in 6–10 min. If $PaCO_2 > 60$ and apneic then +. If apnea test inconclusive, then do a full gain EEG or a transcranial Doppler.
  - *Death note*: VS, CNS (pupil, GCS), $ETCO_2$, tox? asystole in 2–3 leads, lividity, rigor, warm and dead

■ **Death Telling**
  CA Law AB2565 requires waiting "reasonable time" for family to arrive.
  - *Telling*: Family room. Use lay terms (not: MI). If present during code, bring in to "say goodbye." View body, hold child: "Is there someone you'd like me to call?"
  - *"GRIEVE"* (**G**uilt: absolve family; **R**esource: get social work, clergy; **I**ntroduce; **E**vents: give story; **V**alidate: their feelings and loss; **E**mpathize: let them know you are available for question)
  - *By phone*: Only last resort. First ID: name, age, eye color. Use a quiet area, no interruptions.

■ **Organ Donation**
  - *Candidates*: Esp. neurosurgery cases, trauma, CVA, age < 65 and > 4. Need neurologist, PMH-neg.
  - *Dx*: No brainstem reflexes, motor or resp. drive. Nl temp, no drugs, no metabolic.
  - *Tests*: HIV, Hep B/C (do not disqualify though), VDRL, tox screen, TCA level, EEG
  - *Maintain*: Glucose/Na/temp/etc. WNL, keep Hct > 30, pressors as needed +/– thyroid/steroids
  - *Vent goals*: $FiO_2 = 40\%$, $pO_2 > 100$, pCO_2 35–40, pH: 7.35–7.45, TV: 8–10ml/kg, plateau pressure < 30

■ **Palliative Care**
  - Goal is to relieve suffering
  - *Goals*: Treat symptoms (pain, nausea, etc). Provide nutrition and hydration. Provide or assist with emotional and social support. Respect patient's wishes and autonomy.
  - *Benefits*: Cost savings, patient comfort, and autonomy, realistic expectations
  - *Consider*: Law states must inform patient/family about palliative care options. Involving religious leader

■ **DNR and Physician Order for Life-Sustaining Treatment (POLST) Forms**
  - *Meaning*: DNR does not mean do not treat or treat less aggressively. It means no treatment if dead. Nevertheless, people who are DNR often receive less care than is appropriate. Each proposed intervention should have informed consent or refusal from patient or family.
  - *DNR form*: Four things: signed by MD, dx, terminal Px, ID the patient. An MD who knows patient and family may be better at end-of-life decisions than a DNR form.
  - *Death note*: VS, CNS (pupil, GCS), $ETCO_2$, tox? asystole in two to three leads, lividity, rigor, warm, and dead
  - *Physician Order for Life-Sustaining Treatment (POLST)*: Pink sheet specifying level of care desired. Meant to complement not replace an Advance Directive. California law AB3000 requires MDs to honor the POLST form and protects us legally.

CALIFORNIA STATE AND FEDERAL LAW

HEALTH INSURANCE PORTABILITY AND ACCOUNTABILITY ACT (HIPAA)

■ **Do**: Discuss any uncertainties with your hospital's privacy officer. Discuss patient health information with those who have a legitimate need to know. Release one-word condition and general location to others (unless o/w requested not to). Condition: Good, fair, serious, critical, undetermined (not yet seen by MD), deceased; Location: hospitalized, released (treated and released)

■ **Do Not**: Do not put health info in regular trash, ever. Shred it. Don't have loose lips. Do not discuss health information with co-workers, friends, or even family without consent. NO specific health information. NO when's and specific where's (except to family). DO NOT print or take medical records home without permission of hospital privacy officer.

■ **Be Quiet**: Speak softly when discussing private issues and while dictating (use separate room if possible). Be especially careful with regards to patients waiting in a hallway bed.

■ **Computers**: Never share your password. Don't use others' log-ons. Do not e-mail patient info. Always log-off when finished. Access records only on a need-to-know basis.

■ **Photography**: Prior written consent is required for images with patient identifiers (face, tattoo, name, etc.). Prior written consent is recommended for all photography, especially if plan to publish. Written consent may be required by hospital for all photos of patients, employees, and visitors. Each hospital has internal policy on medical photography with consent forms to go in chart. Consent is also required for photographing hospital employees. For more questions, refer to your state hospital association consent manual.

■ **Family**: Do not discuss medical issues with family unless patient has authorized it. This includes discussing medical issues with the patient when others are in the room. Always ask the patient if he or she would prefer privacy.

■ **Sensitive**: Sensitive info includes behavioral and psych, drugs and EtOH, HIV and communicable diseases

■ **Police**: In general, honor a valid search warrant. If unsure, consult with med-record or legal dept.

■ **Fines**: Hospital may be fined up to $25,000 per patient affected and $250,000 per incident per California state law. California SB-541: Requires hospitals to report privacy breaches to the patient and the dept. of health w/in 5d. California AB-211: Office of Health Information and Integrity can investigate MDs, RNs, etc. State can fine individuals $2500 to $250,000 if they sought financial gain with illegal data. The Office of Health Information and Integrity also may recommend that the relevant licensing board conduct an investigation.

MINORS

■ **Emancipated**: Law varies by state: in California: pregnant, age > 15, and live separately or in army

■ **Behavioral**: Can hold minor against will by parental request for behavioral issues if not emancipated

■ **Abuse**: CPS give authority to hold a minor. If parent threatening to staff, can call police or let them go then call CPS and police.

■ **Parents**: If parent tries to take child who needs care, call police and CPS. Consider a court order. You can get sued for restraining the parent.

■ **Court Order**: NOT needed for emergency care, only for ongoing care without parental consent. May use to give blood to a minor when parents refuse.

■ **Child Protective Services (CPS)**: If parents refusing necessary care, call CPS and police immediately. Inquire about holding child. Parents saying "I'll see my doctor tomorrow" may be a lie.

MANDATORY REPORTING

- **General:** You are required to report your suspicion and you don't need to be certain.
- **Protection:** Immunity for the reporting physician against lawsuit for the report.
- **Forms:** 5 separate forms for Animal bite, TB, STD's, HIV, and other.
- **Elder or Child Abuse:** You are required to report your suspicion and you don't need to be certain.
- **Assault:** Crimes of violence.
- **Syncope:** Report any lapse of consciousness. "Do not drive until cleared to by your doctor or specialist."
  - *Examples*: Sleep apnea, Sz, brain tumor, dementia, narcolepsy, DM, syncope, etc. (rules vary by state)
- **Tarasoff:** If a patient threatens to harm a specific person, you have a duty to warn them.
- **CMS:** Events: Air embolism, blood incompatibility, pressure sores, catheter associated infections, falls, post-CABG mediastinitis, post-procedure retained foreign object.
- **Domestic Violence**: Mandatory reporting in California, Colorado, Kentucky, New Hampshire, Rhode Island, New Mexico. Document all injuries using body map and photograph if possible.
  - *Rx*: Call law enforcement and social work. Shelter. National Hotline: (800) 799–7233. Assure safety of patient and any children at home. Consider admission if no other options.
  - *Risks*: Pregnant, depression; harm, threat; firearm? safe return?
  - *Sexual assault*: Call police. If minor refuses exam, then no exam.

PATIENTS IN POLICE CUSTODY

- **Contraband:** Do not search for contraband unless court order or patient gives consent in writing or two MDs declare that contraband is medically life threatening
- **Court Order**: Rare. Call hospital legal services. MD should be immune from civil and criminal charges
- **Blood Draw**: Federal law states blood cannot be drawn without consent if patient competent. For blood alcohol, document; only soap and water was used to prep the skin.
- **Charting**: Use "alleged" or "probable" or "patient states" liberally to avoid being subpoenaed to testify.
- **Convict**: May refuse medical care, rectal exam; but then cannot insist on being medically cleared. Some say don't Rx convict against will even if court order without hospital legal council.
- **Battery**: Touching without consent; but if "patient confused, not lucid; family agrees" use implied consent
- **Sexual Assault**: Call police. If minor refuses exam, then no exam.
- **Abuse?:** Immunity for the reporting physician against lawsuit for the report

SECTION 5 ■ RISK MANAGEMENT, MED-LEGAL, AND BILLING

PATIENT INTERACTIONS

"If you do not like the behavior of another person, change your behavior."
—unknown

■ **Patient and Family Interactions**

- *Patients*: LISTEN. Never refer to a patient in pejorative terms. Crush with kindness; apologize. Treat each patient like family. Err in way patient suffers least. Make a good first impression. Philosophy of YES; anticipate what they want. Don't get angry. It only wastes time. Patients remember the way you made them feel, not how smart you were. Don't speculate when it's better to wait for more data. Don't conceal information. Don't blame others; it won't protect you and you may be dragged into a lawsuit.

- *Satisfaction*: No. 1 predictor of patient satisfaction is physician's nonverbal communication skills.

- *Professional*: Be warm, explain, spend time. Be trustworthy. Put patient's interest first. Give accurate time estimates. YES: Don't explain "we're busy"; they won't understand. Just say yes.

  "Care" (**C**oncentration: Focus on your patient, limit distractions; **A**cknowledgment: If patients are waiting a long time, offer explanations; **R**espect: Introduce yourself by name and title; close the curtain/door for privacy; **E**mpathy, **C**ompassion: Cure sometimes, care always. Hold hands when appropriate)

- *Don't*: Don't delay treatment, don't have lab delays, don't give telephone advice. Don't be judgmental. The less you like a patient, the nicer you should be.

- *Do*: Be nice, listen, make eye contact, sit, close door, involve patient in decisions, call PMD. Always talk to the spouse/family. Explain, apologize, fix problem. Give consistent messaging. Changes can confuse patients. Practice expectation management: give them a realistic idea of how long it will actually take. Patients sue for money > accountability > an explanation of error; didn't meet patient and PMD expectations. Worry: Patient has unreasonable expectations, writing everyone's name, asks to see person in charge. Patient who threatens to sue usually bluffing. Tell them you will document their behavior.

- *Family*: Always talk to family if possible, especially for ACI, informed consent, AMA. Family is a safety net and involving them may prevent a bad outcome or a lawsuit.

- *Expectations*: Make sure they have realistic expectations of timing and outcome.

- *Complaints*: Always listen and address professionally. If you don't, a lawyer will.

■ **Press-Ganey Scores and Expectation Management**

- *Waiting*: Perceived (not actual) waiting time is the most important variable in patient satisfaction. Let them know how long things will take. Overestimate wait times. Explain delays. Helps: Symptoms treated, delays explained, realistic expectations given, patient has company or TV.

- *Reassure*: Reduces anxiety; expresses empathy

- *Solutions*: Explain what can and cannot be accomplished in the ED.

- *Work-ups*: Find out what they are worried about or what they expect, especially in confusing cases.

- *Dying patient*: Ask, "What were you hoping we could do?"

STAFF INTERACTIONS

■ Staff Interactions: Nurses, PMDs, and Consultants

- *All staff*: Thank them, especially for a job well done. Show appreciation.
- *Nurses*: Are a critical part of the team. If you share the plan of care, they can better watch your back. Treat with respect. LISTEN, communicate clearly, and be consistent. Eye contact. Questions: Don't always feel you are being challenged when nurses question your orders. Often they need to know to give report, are curious, or need an explanation for the patient. Sometimes they are double-checking, which is important for patient safety. Thank them whenever they double-check a med order: "Thanks for watching my back." Wants: They want to know you are approachable and working hard.
- *Consultants*: Bad to be talked out of something on the phone. Have them come in. Trust your instincts and gut feelings.You are the patient's advocate. If you do not know what a sick patient has, get a consultation (or two). If you do not agree with consulting MD's care or recommendations, get another opinion. Document number of calls, time of calls, discussion, and ETA of consultant.

■ Coordinating Care: When Multiple MDs Are Involved in Care

- *Take charge*: The attending and ER doctor are in charge of coordinating care. Be certain there is clear communication as to who will be responsible for what.
- *Mix-ups*: Ensure that all MDs give the patient a similar message and have a coordinated plan of care. If there is a complication, everyone should give a similar explanation to avoid suspicion. Verbally warn other members of the team if there is a complaint, complication, status change.
- *Consults*: If the patient requests one, you should arrange it. Document consultant's time of arrival or ETA.
- *Dispos*: Avoid telling a patient they will be admitted until consulting PMD. It is best to make a joint decision with the PMD so patient confidence is maintained. Documenting that another MD is responsible for poor practice does not protect you. If you don't advocate for patient, it increases your risk. A unified front is always better. If you and PMD disagree on dispo, consult for a tie-braker or call the chief of staff.

ED SYSTEMS AND CHARTING

■ ED Systems

- *Pros*: D/C vitals, fast triage, good ACI, fast XR, QA system, good nurses and ratios (3:1, registry?), dictated charts, short wait times, no phone advice (previsit first-aid advice OK if keep a log)
- *Consent*: Risks: death, harm, difficult recuperation, infection, bleeding: "patient understands and agrees"
- *Radiology*: Have preliminary read become part of permanent record because final report often differs
- *Event form*: Unexpected death, procedure comps, upset patient/family, fall in ED, incorrect med given, etc.
- *Admits*: Holding orders not recommended, but if done, copy as "telephone orders" from admitting MD; any holding orders should have an expiration time

■ Test Results

- *X-ray*: Missed nodules that become cancer are a legal risk. Tell patient and PMD and give patient a copy to take with them.
- *Blood*: Don't order tests that won't come back before discharge unless PMD has taken responsibility, e.g., PSA, TSH, blood cultures.

■ Email

- *Pros*: Convenience. Can use medical record numbers to improve confidentiality.
- *Cons*: Discoverable. If kept in the realm of Quality Assurance it is protected.

■ Charting

- *Plaintiff's lawyer*: "Sloppy in charting is sloppy in practice." BE CONCISE.
- *Charting*: "EMT/Triage/Nurses' notes reviewed" and sign them. Do a complete H&P. Note pertinent negatives. Chart should be internally consistent. If H&P is incomplete, you will lose! i.e., bilateral BP, listen for bruits, pulsatile mass. "ED course reviewed with nurse." Always document a re-exam on long stays and re-vitals. Time: Orders, phone calls; how many times consultant was called and discussion. Chart how you involved family. Chart decision-making process. Chart reason for delays.
- *Consistency*: Diagnosis, treatment, and disposition fit with charting of H&P and labs.
- *Legibility*: Very important
- *Changes*: Never alter chart; date, time, and sign additions/corrections. Dictate addendum. Line and write "error." If inappropriately altered may cause case to be lost.

- *Scripts*: Patient notified of impaired driving: antihistamine, narcotic, antiemetic: always warn patient. Avoid narcotics in patients with uncertain dx, especially avoid sending home with narcotics for more than 12–24 hr.
- *After care*: "Patient was counseled on diagnosis or lack thereof, treatment, activity restrictions, reasons to return to the ED and need for follow up care. Verbal and printed after care were provided. Prescriptions were written for _____. All questions were answered."
- *Vitals*: Abnormal discharge vitals are very important. Be sure all vitals are normal or explained.

■ Do's

- *Be accurate*: Don't make assumptions; try to describe as objectively as possible in record.
- *Be brief*: Less is more. Wordy responses are more likely to be misunderstood or trigger suspicion. Wordy charts are more likely to give plaintiff's attorney material on which to build a case.
- *Be complete*: Juries want to see that the doctor was thorough. Document reasoning if not obvious. Complete H&P. Consult liberally and document it.
- *Consistency*: Your records should be consistent with the nurses' and any consultants'. Inconsistencies give a lawyer a chance to pit providers against each other.
- *Warn patient*: Document warnings given to patient: "Explained risks, with emphasis on _____."
- *Give ACI*: Document given printed and verbal: "Patient counseled on the diagnosis and level of certainty, treatment, and side effects, reasons to return to the ER with emphasis on _____, and need to call their doctor tomorrow for further advice and care."
- *Others*: Document noncompliance. Think carefully before you explain a complication.
- *Consults*: Read and respond to recommendations or document a good reason why not.
- *Updating*: Notify patients/family about delays (overestimate them) and abnormal and normal findings.
- *Apologize*: Apologize for waits. Apologize for errors. Be sincere.
- *See all*: Even if PMD seeing or going straight to another part of hospital, see them. You can be sued for a patient you "should" have known about.
- *Make chart*: If there is no chart, there is no malpractice insurance coverage.
- *Recheck*: Always recheck patient at dispo. and document it.
- *Pass-ons*: Introduce patient to new MD. (See Section 4: Diagnoses, Dispositions, and Laws on pages 101–112)
- *Discussions*: Chart discussions with patients and consultants including risks/benefits of treatment options.

■ Don'ts

- *Don't presume*: It's better to wait for more information than to offer a premature opinion. Say, "I don't want to speculate until I have more information." If pressured, "My hunch is...." Mixed messages may confuse patient and lead to distrust. They don't hear the "maybes." It is even worse if different opinions come from multiple MDs, so ask what they've already been told.
- *Don't be defensive*: Document what you observed; avoid defensive speculation. When documenting error, stay concise and objective. Entries should reflect patient care only. Resist the temptation to explain or argue your case in the record. Documentation should be for the PATIENT'S benefit, not MD defense. Avoid blaming/criticizing others; it will just pull you into a case and rarely protects you.
- *Don't be negative*: Avoid negative comments about the patient or their possible ulterior motives. Avoid comments that might lead a jury to think you didn't take the patient seriously. You might say instead that you are unable to find objective basis for the symptoms. You might say the history may not be reliable and state the reasons why. Don't reveal your frustration; instead show patience and understanding. Don't speculate about the care given by others; you were not there at the time; say you can't speculate.
- *Don't alter notes*: Altered or defensive medical records will lose their credibility and imply guilt. The chart and especially late entries should be limited to information that improves patient care. Lawyers may use late entries to discredit physician. Missing records may also imply guilt. If you need to make a change or addendum for patient safety, date, time, and sign. Arguing your case in the record is like testifying without legal counsel.
- *Don't ignore your patients*: If a patient has a complaint/symptom/concern, always acknowledge it, even if it is not relevant. Do not appear callous, disinterested, or arrogant—at least take a look. If you don't have time to address a concern, let them know when you will.
- *Don't hide facts*: If there was a complication, explain it. Don't hide it or avoid the patient. Disclose errors. Put disclosure in medical record. If not done, statute of limitations for discovery not set.
- *Don't delay care*: If patient sent to ED to be seen by PMD, see them anyway. If they refuse, document warning. If patient does not get a medical screening exam, and you are sued, you will lose.

ERRORS, COMPLICATIONS, AND MORE

■ Why People Sue

- *Anger*: Insufficient explanation, lack of warning, being ignored, discourtesy, rough handling; no follow through
- *Desire to*: Hold healthcare providers accountable, prevent similar injury to others, be compensated

■ Dealing with Errors

- *Do*: Inform patient/family what happened, why, and how it happened, and what you're going to do to fix it. Inform patient/family how you will prevent it from happening to others. Document disclosure in record so statute of limitations is set.
- *Don't*: Don't say that it was your fault. Don't blame someone else. Don't submit a bill for care that is required to correct an error. Inform the family of this.

■ Dealing with Complications

- *Don't delay*: Speak with patient as soon as possible to avoid seeming callous or unconcerned.
- *Explanation*: If a patient has a complication, explain it in a concise and factual manner. Omit blame or how careful you were. Don't minimize the complication.

■ Duty to Third Parties

- *Tarasoff*: If a patient threatens to harm a specific person, you have a duty to warn them.
- *Driving*: If a patient is prescribed sedating meds such as antiemetics, antihistamines, narcotics, etc., you must warn them not to drive, etc., or you could be held liable for the life they take.

■ Litigation Threat

- *Lawyers*: If you're not a hospital employee, consult your lawyer before speaking with hospital attorney.
- *Careful*: Limit what you say and write.
- *Reports*: Incident reports are nondiscoverable in most states if you do not refer to them in the record.
- *Products*: Do not discard a defective product. Save it and give to risk manager.

■ Prevention and Documentation

- *Addendums*: Do not do anything to a chart without timing, signing, and dating the late entry.
- *Perception*: Perception of care and communication with patient and family are sometimes more important than actual care.

■ Ethics: Principles of Proper Conduct for Given Circumstances

- *Autonomy*: Respecting the patient's right to make medical decisions
- *Beneficence*: Decisions based on helping the patient
- *Nonmaleficence*: Decisions based on avoiding harm to the patient
- *Deontology*: Decisions based on religious precepts
- *Utilitarianism*: Decisions based on what is good for the population as a whole
- *Assistance*: Social work, ethics committee

MALPRACTICE INSURANCE

■ **Read It**: Read the declaration page at least, better the whole contract
■ **Nose**: Coverage for cases prior to start of contract; uncommon
■ **Tail**: Coverage for cases filed after you leave a job; find out how many years covered
■ **Uncovered**: EM malpractice is different than other types. Charge is per chart. No chart = no coverage. You are uncovered for advice to friends, coworkers, or family, especially if you write a script. You are uncovered for volunteer work unless this was prearranged in writing by carrier.

GOOD SAMARITAN LAW

■ **Covers**: Emergencies with no prearranged doctor–patient relationship, found by chance if no bill sent
■ **Grey Zone**: Nonemergencies, if you accept payment or even a gift, even from a 3rd party (airline)
■ **No Coverage**: Advice to friends, coworkers, colleagues or family, especially if you write a script

SUBPOENAS, DEPOSITIONS, AND CONSULTING (WHERE YOU ARE NOT A DEFENDANT)

■ **Subpoena**: Don't ignore these. Call in a timely fashion. Say you don't remember the case. Tell them you will not provide free expert testimony and only will verify the chart. Notify attorney prior to testimony that you expect payment for any opinion offered.
■ **Deposition**: If you receive notice that a lawyer would like to take your deposition, notify director and carrier. Malpractice carrier may want to assign you an attorney.
■ **Consulting**: Notify your director to avoid potential conflicts. Be sure you do not become an advocate. Only give the most objective testimony. ACEP has been sanctioning MDs for false testimony. The way you conduct yourself could affect your job. Don't use medical center space or resources. Groups: Expert medical witnesses, forensic, TASA

NOTICE OF INTENTION TO SUE OR "BEING SERVED"

■ **The Chart**: Do not add to or alter chart. It WILL be discovered and used against you. Instead, make notes to yourself or "to my lawyer" and date them, but keep any such notes SEPARATE from medical record.
■ **Actions**: Contact your director and malpractice carrier immediately. There is urgency. Don't contact patient once you have been given notice. Can make notes to self.
■ **Discussions**: Don't discuss case with others except during peer review. They might be deposed. Do not contact plaintiff. Such action could result in criminal charges of intimidation. In general it's safe to talk to your spouse.
■ **Resources**: Risk management, www.mdmentor.com

ARBITRATION

■ **General**: Various formulations; often three judges or judge and two lawyers
■ **Pros**: Quicker, cheaper, lower awards, no punitive damages
■ **Cons**: Chance of defense verdict = 50% (compare to 75% in a trial case), no right of appeal

CHOOSING THE RIGHT ATTORNEY

■ **Basics**: For malpractice must show all four of: duty, breech of duty (standard of care), harm, causation
■ **The Lawyer**: You have input into the choice of the lawyer that represents you. You do not have to accept the assigned lawyer, but you should meet with them first. Ask the lawyer if he or she has defended anyone you know. Ask colleague for advice or referral.
■ **Experience**: Find out if attorney is a partner, their win/loss ratio, and experience with similar cases.
■ **Settling**: Insurance company cannot settle without your permission. Settling is a loss for you. Find out what percent of cases your lawyer settles. Settling makes it harder to get a job in the future.
■ **Conflicts**: If the same company is representing your hospital, get a different attorney. Insist. Hospital will do what's in its best interest, not yours. Tell them there is a conflict of interest and put it in writing.
■ **National Practitioner Data Bank**: Notified of any settlement or verdict where money in any amount is given to a plaintiff. Info available to hospitals, insurance carriers, etc., but not to public. Furthermore, the state medical board is notified if amount exceeds a certain dollar value (ex.: $30,000 in California). If you end up on list, it can make malpractice more expensive and prevent you from getting hired.

DEPOSITIONS

- *Basics*: Intended for discovery and clarification of facts; used to bully witness and form strategy. Under oath and becomes part of legal record. Prepare for it carefully. OK to ask for a break.

■ **Deposition Do's**

- Body position: Torso straight; hands on the table with fingers linked. Use preparation expert. Wait a second before answering. Gives you time to think and your lawyer time to object. Listen carefully to questions. Don't confuse memory questions with customary practice ones.

- Keep answers short. They may be used against you. The less you say the better: "yes;" "no." You'll have the opportunity to give the answers you want when your lawyer asks in court. If record is incomplete, you may say what your usual custom and practice is for situation. Try to answer concisely. If you do not recall, say so. Be polite, concise, and professional.

- Make them work for answers. They may forget to ask things. Yes or no is a good answer. Ask for clarifications of compound questions or if a long statement precedes a question. Say, "I don't understand that question so I can't answer it"; "Would you like to rephrase it?" Take breaks during deposition. Recharge and get advice from your lawyer on how you're doing. When requesting clarification of a question, try to be helpful more than evasive. When asked to interpret tests, go into detail (i.e., the MCHC on the CBC).

■ **Deposition Don'ts**

- Give scientific references: They will be read and used against you. It helps the plaintiff.
- If asked if anything is a reliable authority, answer "no." Instead, cite "professional experience," which doesn't help plaintiff and can't be used against you.
- Be humorous or sarcastic. Don't try to make the attorney look foolish.
- Mention how "busy" it was. It buys no solace and opens you up to more risk.
- Teach them medicine. In a trap question, just answer, "that is not accurate."
- Lose your cool. Plaintiff lawyer may try to get you to lose your temper to size you up.

■ **Experts**: You may attend the deposition of the plaintiff's expert. This may soften their statements.

■ **Post-Depo**: Read deposition transcript for errors and correct them.

TRIAL AND CROSS EXAMINATION

■ **Appearance**: Attend every day with your spouse if possible, even if you will not be on the stand. Look respectable but not too fancy. Try to attend even days you are not on stand. Don't dress too fancy.

■ **Plaintiffs**: May ask the same question over and over. May ask bad questions: Say, "I don't understand that question so I can't answer it"; "Would you like to rephrase it?" If interrupted by lawyer, look at jury and say, "Do you mind if I finish my answer?"

■ **Replying**: If question is vague, double negative, etc., respond with request for clarification. Pause before answer; just the facts; answer to jury (eye contact). Don't use absolutes; "more likely than not" is good. Convey to jury that you are careful, competent, and compassionate. Don't lie. It will hurt you. If you feel so, you may state you feel a question is "beyond the scope of this inquiry."

■ **Do's and Don'ts**

- *Do*: Look at jury when answering question. Stay cool: Prosecutor may tray to get you to lose your temper so you look bad; DON'T. Know your deposition so they can't twist it to use it against you.

- *Don't*: Sound condescending, even if insulted. Parry with lawyer. Lie. Fidget. Answer unclear questions. Do things jury might dislike, such as rolling your eyes.

■ **Texts**: Don't say any text is authoritative or they will use it against you. Say "I base my opinion on everything I have read and my clinical experience."

EXCESSIVE AWARDS

■ **Expose**: If other parties have already settled, be sure the jury knows the dollar amounts. They will likely lower the remaining settlement awarded.

■ **Appeal**: If award is excessive, appeal. Plaintiff may prefer a smaller award now than to wait for appeal.

EXPERT WITNESSES

■ **Ethics**: Expert should function as an agent of the court, not of a particular party. Testimony should be based on facts and medicine, not on allegiance to a particular side. In reality, however, this rarely occurs.

■ **Daubert Challenge**: Use against plaintiff's expert if they give bogus testimony.

■ **Reaffirmation**: Plaintiff's expert should be asked to sign ACEP's expert witness reaffirmation statement.

■ **Censure**: Ask the expert if they have ever been censured.

BILLING

"You make a living by what you get. You make a life by what you give"

—Winston Churchill

TABLE 5.1.   Billing Levels for Emergency Department Charting

Billing		Elements Needed					
Coding Levels	Charges	HPI	PMH/FH/SH	ROS	Exam	Tests / RX	Example
Level 2	$57–224	1	0	1	2	0–1/OTC	sunburn
Level 3	$104–396	1	0	1	2	1–2/script	ankle
Level 4	$159–696	4	1 of 3	2	5	3+ /IM, IV fluids	asthma
Level 5	$250–985	4	2 of 3	10	8	4+ /IV, 2+ nebs	chest pain
Critical Care	$337–1200	# min 0		0		?	ICU, on heparin
	Time blocks: 40 (30–74 min), 80 (75–104 min), 120 (105–134 min)						
	Be sure to document reassessments and responses to therapy.						
Documentation	ROS, EKG, and pulse ox interpretation, critical care time, HPI with ≥ four qualifiers						
Procedures	Document indication and how tolerated. Don't forget: CPR						
	Fracture care	Identify bone and exact location; procedure note for reductions					
	Sedation	"protocol followed" pulse ox and monitor per protocol					
	Laceration repair	Simple: trim and clean; intermed: multilayer, debride; complex: 3 layer					

MORE POSSIBLE EXAMPLES

■ **Level 1:** Suture removal, dT only

■ **Level 2:** OM or sore throat without fever, URI, abrasion/contusion w/o x-ray, rash, sunburn. No Rx. Sprain/strain, laceration w/o repair, insect bite, toothache, dermatitis, impetigo, med refill

■ **Level 3:** UTI, bronchitis, minor trauma with xray, back sprain, SOB or allergic reaction w/o testing. Head injury w/o CT, acute pain, abscess, fever > 100.5, prescription.

■ **Level 4:** Chest pain, trauma minor, abdo/back pain, head injury c CT, depression, asthma, vag bleed. Multiple injuries, advanced imaging, dehydration w/ labs and IV infusion/meds. Pneumonia, SOB with testing, fracture/dislocation, syncope

   ● *Orders*: 3 or more tests

■ **Level 5:** CP, MI, resp distress, CHF, OD, seizure, cardiac arrest, status asthmaticus, sepsis, SBO. Most admits/transfers, cardiac w/u, advanced procedures

   ● *Orders*: ABG, blood culture, transfusion, >2 respiratory treatments, hypovolemia, IV medication/fluids

■ **Critical Care:** AMS, severe dyspnea, AMI, acute CVA, unstable vitals, sepsis, AAA, DKA, transfusions

   ● *Possibly*: Possible ACS, dysrhythmia, hypotension, GI Bleed, TIA/CVA, major trauma, peritonitis. Ectopic, severe SOB, serious OD, HLOC transfers, positive head CT, CHF, HTN emergency. Serious electrolyte problem (K >6.5 or <2.5)

   ● *Time*: Includes test interpretation, history from family/EMS/records/PMD, consult, documenting

HMOs AND DENIAL OF CARE

■ **IMR**: Independent medical review
■ **Purpose**: Patients who have been denied treatment by HMO get decision reviewed by impartial doctor.
■ **Method**: First participate in plan's own grievance process, then e-mail helpline@dmhc.ca.gov

LOST REVENUE: COMMON SOURCES AND DOCUMENTATION RECOMMENDATIONS

■ **Pulse Ox**: Requires the reading AND your interpretation (adequate, low, normal, etc.)
■ **EKG**: Need to comment on rate, rhythm, and at least one other element as well as your interpretation
■ **Ortho**: "Splint in good position, distally neuro-vascular status intact"; "supportive" or "restorative" splinting/strapping, WHO placed splint and a post-placement check. RVUs for restorative care are higher. Document location of injury in detail.
■ **X-rays**: State the number of views and your interpretation.
■ **Downcodes**: Often 5 to 4 because fewer than 10 systems on ROS or 8 systems on physical exam
■ **Critical Care**: Consider for ICU admits, ACS, or PE, risk of sudden deterioration, high complexity decisions; immediate potential for medical crisis, life-threatening Dx; often not documented; Blocks: 0–74 min, 75–104 min, 105–134 min, 135–164 min. Time in procedures (ETT, CPR, CVC, pacer, EKG read) does NOT count so mention this.
■ **Infusion Rx**: Length of infusion time, meds/fluids infused, supervision, necessity, response, and reassess
■ **Sedation**: Indication, review of H&P, consent, preprocedure assessment form, NPO status, ASA class, meds and doses, complications, post-procedure, monitoring, physician intra-service time
■ **Present on Admission (POA)**: Medicare no longer pays for certain hospital acquired conditions. Be sure to document if bedsores, UTI, etc., were POA, otherwise hospital loses money.

MEDICAL DECISION MAKING

Document it.

■ **General**: Summarize complaint, exam, result interpretation, DDx, and thought processes
■ **History**: Old records reviewed; Hx from family, EMS, or alternate source
■ **Tests**: Tests, results, and your interpretation as well as tests you decided against
■ **DDx**: Diagnoses considered and reasons for and against
■ **Rx**: Meds, procedures; include response; reassessment; observation
■ **Dispo.**: Admit or home; arranged outpatient follow-up or tests arranged can support level 5
■ **Risk Level**: Risks involved; complicating factors and comorbidities
■ **Consults**: Who consulted, recommendation, and your decisions

DIAGNOSTIC TERMINOLOGY

■ **Order**: List diagnoses in order of severity or seriousness
■ **Be Specific**: Qualify diagnoses with appropriate modifiers such as type, location, etc.
■ **Acuity**: Qualify with terms such as "acute", "chronic," or "acute on chronic"; Terms: acute, severe, sudden, or unstable may increase billing; mild, minor, possible, chronic, probably, or rule out are terms likely to decrease billing

FRAUD

■ **Procedures**: Must say who did procedure (you, resident, tech, surgeon, etc.) and if supervised by you
■ **Billing**: Can only bill for services that are performed, documented, and medically necessary; cannot bill for services not provided; cannot rebill—must refund credit balances
■ **Kickbacks**: For referrals, etc., can be money, cheaper rent, discounts, etc.
■ **Patient Fraud**: Patient and doctor fake disease of injury to collect money from insurance
■ **National Stark Law**: No self-referral; cannot invest in a company you refer to

SECTION 6 ■ ACADEMICS, TEAMWORK, AND WELL-BEING

MEDICAL LITERATURE BASICS

STUDY METHODS, DESIGN TYPES, AND CONSIDERATIONS

- **Experimental**: Subjects are randomly assigned to groups and results measured afterwards. Ask, randomized? Blinded? Control group (is it valid)? Population? Conflicts of interest?
- **Observational**: Cross-sectional: Measure exposure and outcome simultaneously.
  - *Case-control*: First identify disease, then look for prior exposure; odds ratios
  - *Cohort study*: First identify exposure, then follow for onset of disease; relative risk
- **Literature Review**: There are two types. Systematic is more rigorous than Narrative.
  - *Narrative*: Author uses articles they found and chose to include.
  - *Systematic*: Explicit search strategy used to choose and include or exclude articles; articles are weighted based on quality; may include performing a meta-analysis
- **Population**: What is the population studied? i.e.: chest pain: definite dz, probable dz, Sx only? Number Needed to Harm (NNTH) is always the same but NNT varies with prevalence. If only 50% actually have the dz, the NNT ↑ two-fold. Less benefit but same risk
- **Confounders**: Associations between treatment and outcome possibly due to other factors. Factors that happen to be more common in the experimental than the control group.

COMMON BIASES

- **Comparison Bias**: Control group is inappropriate; possibly they get subtherapeutic dose of competitor
- **Hawthorne Effect**: Process of studying something causes improved medical care and better results. They know they're being watched, so they behave differently.
- **Incorporation Bias**: The results of the test being studied are used as part of the gold standard (unblinded)
- **Observational Bias**: Observers not blinded; result recording process not standardized
- **Publication Bias**: Negative studies are often not published; meta-analyses magnify this bias. Of preregistered studies, a minority are currently published. The percentage is even lower for drug company sponsored studies. This shows how greatly distorted the medical literature is.
- **Recall Bias**: Patients with the disease may better recall what they think was the proximate cause. Patients without the disease may have poorer recall of a potential causal event.
- **Selection Bias**: Population studied is selected differently from the reader's patient population. Can be due to geography, insurance, race, but is most notable in referral populations.
- **Spectrum Bias**: Early/mild disease presentation is less likely to have a positive test result.
- **Sponsorship Bias**: Industry-sponsored studies FAR more likely to be positive than nonindustry studies. THIS IS HUGE: Be very skeptical about any sponsored study.
- **Workup Bias**: Some patients never get a gold standard test (Dx'd only by the test being studied).

WAYS TO FOOL THE READER

- **Data**: Distortion, not reporting missing data, ignoring outliers, not reporting side effects
- **One Sided**: Not publishing negative studies, not referencing contradictory studies, undisclosed conflicts
- **Results**: Post-hoc analysis

RESULTS REPORTING

■ **Likelihood Ratio**: Positive likelihood ratios: > 10 is good; > 5 is helpful; < 5 is not helpful. Negative likelihood ratios: < 0.1 is good; < 0.5 is helpful; > 0.5 is not helpful.

■ **Odds Ratio**: Odds of an outcome in treatment group versus odds of the outcome in the control group.

■ **Absolute Benefit**: Gives the absolute benefit. Compare to relative benefit.

■ **Relative Benefit**: Drug companies often report relative benefits. A decrease in mortality from 2% to 1% will be called a 50% decrease rather than 1%.

■ **Number Needed to Treat (NNT)**: A better way to give results related to absolute benefit. Avoids "inflation" or relative benefit reporting.

■ **Number Needed to Harm (NNTH)**: Related to absolute magnitude of harm.

■ **Test Characteristics**: How well a test performs. T = True, F = False, P = Positive, N = Negative.

- *Sensitivity*: How sensitive is a test when it is negative. Sensitivity = TP/(TP + FN).
- *Specificity*: How specific is a test when it is positive. Specificity = TN/(TN + FP).
- *Negative Predictive Value (NPV)*: True negatives out of total negatives. NPV = TN/(TN + FN). Looks better than sensitivity if prevalence of disease low. This is a favorite trick of many authors to make their test look good.
- *Positive Predictive Value (PPV)*: True positives out of total positives. PPV = TP/(TP + FP). Looks worse than specificity if prevalence of disease low; looks better than specificity if prevalence of disease is high (a rare case).

ADDITIONAL IMPORTANT CONCEPTS TO UNDERSTAND WHEN INTERPRETING STUDIES

■ **Composite Endpoint**: Makes it more likely that at least one endpoint will show positive results by chance; effect = a bigger target. The more endpoints the more you should beware.

■ **Early Termination**: Be suspicious if drug company sponsored; motives for an early stop often suspect.

■ **External Validity**: Are the results generalizable to the patients you see? Most studies use high acuity, low comorbidity patients; when compared to average population, this increases benefit and decreases death.

■ **Meta-Analysis**: Many pitfalls, including publication bias

■ **Post-Hoc Analysis**: Aka subgroup analysis, data dredging, data torture, data snooping Analyzing (-) data by breaking into subgroups to find a subgroup with (+) results. If you have enough subgroups, then just by chance, some will end up looking good. This is NOT acceptable for forming conclusions. It may be used to generate a hypothesis only.

■ **Relative Risk**: Drug companies often report RELATIVE benefits. A decrease in mortality from 2% to 1% will be called a 50% decrease rather than 1%.

■ **Significance**: Is the effect both statistically and clinically significant?

■ **Spin**: Pay attention to potential conflicts of interest and who funded the study. Consider NOT reading the discussion because this is where the spin mostly occurs.

■ **Straw Man**: Aka faulty comparators. Ask yourself: Is the dose for the competitor right? Did they compare to placebo rather than to the current standard treatment?

■ **Surrogate Markers**: Endpoints measured are not those that matter, but are assumed to relate to them; i.e.: measuring lab or imaging results rather than patient outcome results

TEAMWORK IN THE ED

DOCTORS

■ Goals for Doctors

Make an effort to say "hello," "good-bye," and "thank you"; we all work harder, better, and longer when we feel respected and appreciated.

- *Aftercare*: Include the most important test results so nurse can communicate better with patients. Patients often want to know test results and may not remember what MD told them.

- *Nurses*: When someone is talking to you, let them know you appreciate their input; make eye contact. Acknowledge what they said; say, "thank you" even if you are under stress or swamped. Maintain a professional tone of voice. Nurses often feel they don't receive proper respect. It is better to have to hear the same thing twice than to have nurses not keep you informed. Always involve nurse in the treatment plan, especially if they ask. Communication is key to preventing errors and to ensure timely care. Remember that the nurse is your eyes and ears when you are not there.

- *Patients*: Dispo. ASAP. After the H&P, let patient and family know what to expect. Inform: IV, X-rays, other tests, pain medication, expected time in department, probable disposition. Realize that some patients may be pleasant with the doctor but then be rude with the nurse.

- *Workload*: Before contacting triage about bringing patients back, ask RN if it is OK. If RN staffing is short, possibly MDs could help out by taking vitals, starting lines, etc.

- *BONUS*: Let a person's supervisor know when they do an outstanding job or make a good save. Buy food every once in a while; people appreciate the thought and the nourishment.

■ Dale Carnegie's Wisdom and More*

Don't criticize others; instead assume they are just doing what you would do under similar circumstances. Think about others rather than about yourself. Express your appreciation often. Try to see things from the other person's point of view. Get in the habit of telling other people they are right. Show respect for other's opinions.

*Adapted from Carnegie, D. How to Win Friends and Influence People. Simon & Schuster, 2009.

> "He who travels softly goes far"
> —Chinese proverb

> "Men must be taught as if taught not, and things unknown proposed as things forgot."
> —Alexander Pope

■ Getting Along with Others

- *Patients*: Press-Ganey scores: taking time to explain care, friendliness, providing for comfort, seeing patients in a timely fashion, explaining delays, treating pain, caring. Confidentiality and privacy: Close the curtain, speak softly, but let family in. Hygiene: Wash your hands! And let the patient see it. Complaints: Thank person for taking time to raise concern. Make it a positive experience. Use as a chance for improvement. Be honest and sincere. Don't blame; search for a solution.

- *Nurses*: Be approachable, discuss plan of care, thank them for watching your back.

- *Pass-ons*: Try to have a dispo., try to have finished calls to PMDs, even if tests still pending. Let patient know you are leaving and the plan. Wrap up loose ends whenever possible. Use SBAR: situation, background, assessment, recommendation.

- *Other MDs*: Be careful what you chart about difficult MDs. Don't complain/deride in chart. Be careful how you question another physician's judgement.

NURSES

■ Goals for Nurses

Make an effort to say simple things: "Hello," "good-bye," "thank you"; we all work harder, better, and longer when we feel respected and appreciated.

- *Orders*: Try not to interrupt MD while he or she is writing orders because this is a big source of error.

- *MD stress*: When multiple people need MD simultaneously. Interruptions (part of working in the ED, but try to do it with skill); having to answer the same question from multiple people. Juggling multiple "to-do's" (most common reason MD appears to show lack of attention)

- *Extra mile*: When you are caught up, aid in timely disposition by going one step further than asking, "What is the plan?" Are there missing labs that need to be on the chart? How are the vitals? Is the patient is able to walk, talk, and drink? Make your own assessment.

- *After care instructions*: Circle and read what the doctor typed in freehand on the aftercare sheet.

- *Back-up*: No one is perfect; we all need back-up. Demonstrate patient advocacy by questioning orders that don't make sense and making suggestions to physician if important testing or treatment seems to have been omitted. Good examples include beta-blocker in chest pain, antibiotics delays (more important than the Tylenol), aspirin after negative head CT in TIA/stroke patient (often forgotten), drug levels for seizure meds, coumadin, etc.

■ Tiers of Nursing Care Sophistication

1. Picking up errors in orders such as wrong patient, missed allergy, unnecessary test
2. Updating physician on change in status such as new fever, new vital signs, or worsening pain
3. Symptom management (pain, vomiting, fever)
    - *Safety*: No narcotics, sedatives, or antiemetics except Zofran if driving. Ibuprofen safer, cheaper, and as effective as ketorolac (Toradol)
    - *Be cost effective*: Newer medications cost the most. Antiemetics NOT recommended prophylactically with narcotics.
    - *Fever*: Fever helps to fight infection and is in general beneficial. Give antibiotics if ID is bacterial. Exceptions to not treating: tachycardia, seizure, interferes with evaluation, patient preference.
4. Improve patient flow preparing for dispo. prior to asking MD about it
    - Reconcile tests and have on chart
    - Repeat vitals, esp. if tachycardia or low BP; orthostatics if "weakness" or borderline vitals
    - *Road test*: PO trial if vomiting, trial of ambulation prn
    - *Transportation*: Ride home if getting sedating medications
5. "Reminding" physicians if certain key aspects of care have been omitted. For this, you need to make your own assessment and expected treatment course.
    - *Chest pain*: "MONA" (**M**orphine, **O**xygen, **N**itrates, **A**spirin)
    - *CHF*: Nitrates if BP high, ACE inhibit > Lasix
    - *Pneumonia*: Blood cultures, antibiotics given in less than 4 hr
    - *Wheezing*: Steroids, atrovent, beta agonist, pulse ox
    - *Stroke/TIA*: Aspirin should be ordered if CT shows no bleed
    - *Heparin*: Should have the CBC results back before starting
    - *GI bleed*: Type and screen ordered, proton pump inhibitory (Protonix, Prevacid, Nexium)

CAREER, WELLNESS, AND FINANCE

JOB SEARCH AND INTERVIEWING

■ **Do's**
- Know about the job so you can ask good questions (prepare some). Bring copies of your CV.
- Be ready for tough questions: "Why should we hire you?"; "What are your weaknesses?" Show respect for everyone, even more so if they work in the director's office.

■ **Don'ts**
- Don't criticize prior employers. Avoid any criticism.
- Don't leave a bad impression even if you decide against the job. EM is a small world.

THE JOB

■ **Pay**: Hourly; fee for service: pay of 70% of billing is average
■ **Shifts**: 8 hr or 12 hr? On call? Shifts/month? No. of night shifts and is there extra pay
■ **Benefits**: Malpractice: type, limits. 401K, partnership
■ **Turnover**: Is this an additional position or did someone leave? If someone left, why?
■ **Ancillary**: Patient-to-nurse ratio: > 4:1 is bad. Clerks, EMTs, etc.
■ **Hospital**: On-call panel and does it have holes

PROFESSIONALISM AND KEEPING YOUR JOB

■ **Do's**
- Do be polite.
- Do be a team player: make others, esp. your boss, look good.
- Do network with others.
- Do groom and dress professionally.
- Do take customer satisfaction seriously.
- Do pull your own weight.

■ **Don'ts**
- Don't be a jerk; people prefer likeable but less-skilled coworkers.
- Don't miss deadlines; it's better to under-promise and over-deliver.
- Don't conduct personal business when you're on the clock.
- Don't put anything in an e-mail you don't want your boss to see.
- Don't do anything that could be construed as sexual harassment.
- Don't gossip, tell off-color jokes, or be indiscreet.
- Don't get a number of complaints from patients and/or staff.
- Don't be high maintenance; don't take up your director's time.
- Don't scold or argue with nurses, residents, or anyone who might "report" you.

SEXUAL HARASSMENT: A COSTLY MISTAKE

■ **Definition**: Unwanted sexual advances or visual, verbal, or physical conduct of a sexual nature.
■ **Includes**: Leering, displaying suggestive objects, sexual jokes, touching, blocking movement
■ **How It Is**: You only need to be accused to lose your job. If others are joking, simply walk away.

MEDICAL BOARD INVESTIGATIONS

■ **Triggers:** Complaints, poor record keeping, unethical behavior, negligence
- *Addiction*: Substance abuse, DUI, alcoholism, self-prescribing controlled substances
- *Sex*: Sexual relations with patient or their spouse, sexual comments
- *Theft/lies*: Fraud, stealing from hospital, not reporting criminal record, dishonest expert testimony
- *Scripts*: Excessive prescribing to addicts without exam

HEALTH

- ◼ **Sleep**
  - ● Consistent schedule, dark room, limit caffeine and EtOH, white noise machine, cool bedroom
  - ● Nap before first night shift, but if unable to fall asleep in 20 min, get out of bed
  - ● Do isolated night shifts rather that clustering to avoid resetting internal circadian clock.
  - ● Sunglasses on way home after night shift; very dark room.
  - ● Don't exercise right before sleep.
  - ● Try to keep as consistent a sleep schedule as possible and eat the same times of day.
- ◼ **Diet:** Eat healthy. Take a multivitamin.
- ◼ **Driving:** For the drive home, take a 30-min nap in the call room.
- ◼ **Drugs:** Emergency physicians are at high risk for substance abuse. Don't self treat. Get help from your doctor, your hospital's confidential wellness committee, or the state.
- ◼ **Infection**: Odds ratios for reducing respiratory disease: N95 mask > gown > any mask > gloves > hand washing.
- ◼ **Leisure:** Get adequate exercise; it's good for your heart, your brain, your sleep, and your sanity. Prioritize!

BURNOUT AND QUITTING

- ◼ **Symptoms**: Denial, isolation, anxiety, dread of work, depression, anger at work, addiction, risk taking. Sleep disorders, exhaustion, eating disorders.
- ◼ **Treatment**: Vacation, counseling, social support, gradual reintroduction to work with limited hours
- ◼ **Prevention**: Proper sleep, exercise, and nutrition. Managing stress, sharing stories.
- ◼ **Quitting**: Never quit in the middle of a shift. You could be accused of patient abandonment.

PRESS-GANEY SCORES

- ◼ **Courtesy**
  - ● Introduce self. Eye contact. Shake hands. Wash hands. Sit low. Don't leave while talking. Overcome your biases. Non-verbal behavior. Don't be dismissive or rude. Respect privacy. Don't stand in doorway. Return after an interruption. Show concern and empathy.
- ◼ **Listening**
  - ● Don't ignore any patient concerns, even if they seem trivial. Open ended questions. Avoid interrupting patient. Eye contact. Make patient feel important. Write notes. Summarize history back to patient. Respond empathetically. Don't rush. Ask, "What do you think is the matter and what do you think should be done?" Nod a lot.
- ◼ **Informing**
  - ● Inform patients of test results and planned treatment. Patients often feel forgotten. Explain delays (and overestimate them). Warn of unpleasant treatments, respect confidentiality. Update patient frequently. Educate patient and assess understanding. "Any questions?"
- ◼ **Comfort**
  - ● Treat pain compassionately (make sure they have a ride home). Offer blanket, drink, food… Ask "Is there anything I can do to make you more comfortable?" Show empathy.

THE JOINT COMMISION (TJC) AND SITE SURVEYS

- **Administrators**: _____ COO = _____ CEO = _____ Safety Representative = _____
- **Communication:** Use approved abbreviations, use two patient identifiers, read-back of orders
  - *Hand-offs*: Use "SBAR" (**S**ituation, **B**ackground, **A**ssessment, **R**ecommendations)
- **Fire:** Know where nearest alarm and extinguishers are located; up-to-date fire card/class
  - *"SKATE"* (**S**afety of life, "**K**ontain" fire, **A**ssistance, **T**elephone report, **E**xtinguish if safe)
- **Never 27:** California SB1301: 27 Things that Should **Never** Occur in The Medical Center
  - *5 Surgery*: Wrong part or side, wrong patient, wrong procedure, retained foreign body, unexpected death
  - *3 Devices*: Serious injury from contamination, improper use or function, air embolism
  - *3 Protection*: Infant discharged to wrong person, patient disappearance > 4 hr, suicide attempt
  - *7 Care*: Serious injury from med. error, hemolysis p transfusion, hypoglycemia, or manipulating spine, maternal death in low-risk pregnancy, kernicterus, progression of stasis ulcers
  - *5 Environs*: Serious injury from electric shock, burn, fall, restraints or bedrails, or toxins in oxygen line
  - *4 Criminal*: Provider impersonators, patient abduction, sexual assault, injury from physical assault
- **Privacy:** Close charts, use shredder bins, discuss patient info only with those who need to know
- **Procedures:** If using sedation must conduct and document a presedation assessment
  - *Consent*: Must document informed consent prior to procedure (including LP) or transfusion
  - *Lines*: Use maximal barriers: mask/eye shield, sterile gown, large full body sterile drape on patient, cap; must wash hands for 20 sec or use alcohol cleanser prior to performing procedure.
  - *Time Out*: Confirm correct patient, correct procedure, correct side, correct equipment, correct drugs
- **Safety:** Peds dosing must be per kg and calculations shown
  - *Hygiene*: Wash or sanitizer before and after every patient encounter. Wide sterile barriers for lines
  - *Falls*: Report spilled liquid and torn carpet
  - *Wrist Bands*
    Red: Allergy
    Yellow: Fall Risk
    Purple: DNR
    Blue: Isolation
    Green: Difficult intubation
    Orange: Visitor

ABEM AND THE EMERGENCY MEDICINE CONTINUOUS CERTIFICATION (EMCC)

- **Lifelong Learning Self Assessment (LLSA):** A yearly, 40 question, "open-book" style online test.
  - *Score*: You may take three times (pay only once). Need 85–90% to pass.
  - *Dates*: Tests retired March 31st of the 3rd year after first posted. New test available each April 1st.
- **Continuous Certification Exam (ConCert):** A proctored exam that must be taken every 10 years. The ConCert is given in a national test center. To take ConCert, you must first pass 8 of 10 of the yearly LLSA tests.
- **Assessment of Practice Performance (APP):** Takes effect in 2011. Must attest to participation in two practice improvement programs that meet requirements. Must complete one communication/professionalism activity

FINANCE AND SAVINGS

- **Buying:** Spend less; $1000 you save today may be $10,000 in 20 years
- **Saving:** Prioritize it; do what you need to do to make it happen
- **Deductions:** Pretax earnings into IRAs
- **Schedules**: A: State, home loan, charity, medical, work; B: Interest; C: Business; D: Capital gains/losses
- **Investment:** Start with index funds like SPYDERS or Vanguard. These passive funds outperform most actively managed funds and have low maintenance cost.
- **Asset Protection:** Once you are sued, it is too late. No strategy is foolproof. $$ in an IRA, your 1st home, a trust, spouse/child's name, or an annuity might be protected.
- **FDIC:** Does cover $100,000 per person per bank ($250,000 for IRAs); does NOT cover: stocks, bonds, mutual funds, money market mutual funds
- **SIPC:** Make sure your brokerage firm is SIPC insured: $500,000 per person ($100,000 for cash)

INCORPORATION

- **Pros**: Higher retirement contribution possible ($45,000), more deductions (health, leased car); limits personal liability, shares of stock can be transferred to children, group term life insurance
- **Cons:** Higher social security tax, unemployment tax, need an accountant, set-up cost ($1000+); costs may be higher than benefit if make < $200,000/year
- **Types:** C-corp: The basic type of corporation; S-corp: A C-corp that has elected to have special tax status; this benefit comes with certain restrictions
- **Process**: Choose a state and name, stock, file certificate, write by-laws, hold annual meeting
- **Accounting**: Federal forms: 941, 940-EZ, W2, W3, W4 for each employee; taxes: 1120A, FICA, FUTA; California forms: DE1, DE6, DE88, DE34. Taxes: SDI, ETT, unemployment, income. Also have to do personal income tax.

SOME BASIC INSURANCE NEEDS

- **Car:** Liability is a must; theft and collision not as much so.
- **Disability:** Pays if you can't work. Own occupation better than general. Expensive. Often a 1–3 mon waiting period before it kicks in.
- **Health:** Preferred Provider Organization (PPO): You choose your provider; costs more. Health Maintenance Organization (HMO): You must select from contracted providers; cheaper. Point of Service (POS): In between PPO and HMO.
- **Home:** Homeowner's = dwelling (fire) + liability (someone injured) + property (valuables in house); earthquake or flood extra
- **Life:** Pays your family if you die
- **Malpractice:** For emergency physicians, usually bought by group; no chart = no malpractice insurance. If you give advice or write a script for a friend, you have NO coverage.
- **Umbrella:** Covers liability beyond your other policies; usually at least $1 million

RANDOM THOUGHTS

RULES

■ **For The Internal Medicine Resident**

- *Incidence*: Common things occur commonly.
- *Treatment*: If what you are doing is working, keep doing it. If not, stop. If you don't know what to do, don't do anything.
- *Consults*: If you are stumped, get a consult, but don't let a surgeon get your patient.

■ **For The Surgical Resident**

- *Food*: Eat when you can.
- *Sleep*: Sleep when you can.
- *Pitfalls*: Don't mess with the pancreas.

■ **For The Emergency Medicine Resident**

- *The Four A's*: Availability, Affability, Ability, and Antibiotics
- *Uncertainty*: Don't just do something; stand there.
- *Consultants*: Apologize for disturbing them. Don't turn a disagreement into an argument.
- *Disagreements*: Consider it an opportunity to avoid a mistake. Start by assuming you are wrong (even though you know you are right), then find a common ground to work from. If you can't agree, insist other doctor come in and see the patient.

■ **For Being Pimped: Some Answers**

- *The ABC's*: Always a good answer when asked, "What would you do first?"
- *It depends*: Never give a wrong answer—but it won't prevent the next question.
- *15% or 85%*: Choose one of these when asked a "What percent…" question. Usually you will be close enough. They will be pleased to give you the exact answer.

REBUTTALS TO EVIDENCE-BASED MEDICINE FANATICS

■ **Quip**: Absence of evidence is not evidence of absence.

■ **Science**: A meta-analysis of the use of parachutes to prevent injury during free-falls came to the conclusion that further randomized controlled studies are needed.

OCCAM'S RAZOR

■ **Latin**: Entia non sunt multipicanda praeter necessitatem.

■ **English**: No more things should be presumed to exist than are necessary.

■ **Application**: Explore the simplest explanation first.

■ **EP**: Assume the most serious cause first.

SEEING RED

■ **Red Flag**: A finding that increases suspicion of disease presence or severity

■ **Red Herring**: A smelly fish used by criminals to cover their tracks and lure hounds off of their trail. Used to describe a clinical finding that distracts the clinician from the correct diagnosis.

■ **Red Man**: A patient who is having an adverse reaction to Vancomycin. Rx: Slow the rate.

■ **Red Tide**: An overgrowth of certain dinoflagellates that can contaminate or kill fish. Note: Eating from these waters can cause paralytic shellfish poisoning.

SECTION 7 ■ RESUSCITATION

ADULT RESUSCITATION

CHOKING BASICS
■ **Moving Air:** Encourage patient to cough. For infants, give 5 back slaps and up to 5 chest thrusts.
■ **Gasping:** Heimlich or abdominal thrusts. Give chest thrusts if obese or pregnant.
■ **Collapse:** CPR. Finger sweep only for visible foreign body.

CPR BASICS
■ **Safety:** Nurse should "read back" all verbal orders.
■ **Preparation:** Crash cart, echo/Doppler and NG tube syringe as esophageal or end-tidal CO_2 detector; ask medics Rx so far (volts, epi, atropine, etc.)
■ **Family:** May be present, but best if dedicated staff to be with them and explain proceedings
■ **CPR Ratios:** 30:2 Adults until intubated (then no ratio, just rates); 15:2: Peds; 3:1: Newborn
  ● *Rate/depth:* Adult: RR: 8–10, HR: 100/2"; Age < 8: RR: 20, HR: 100+/1.5"; Age < 1: RR: 20+, HR: 120/1"
■ **Compression:** Rate = 100/min: use beat to BeeGee's song "Staying Alive," full chest recoil
  ● *Preshock:* 200 preshock compressions if down more than 5–10 min.
  ● *Fast and hard:* Push hard, push fast. Use backboard. Change compressor every 2 min. with rhythm check.
  ● *Nonstop:* Avoid compression interruption.
  ● *"Toxins":* 2 min CPR before defib to push out toxins. 2 min CPR p conversion b/c heart still stunned.
  ● *Consider:* Interposed abdominal compressions; Infant: Two thumb compression best
■ **Ventilation:** Bag slower (8–10/min) so don't hyperventilate. Hyperventilation decreases venous return, tissue O_2 delivery (because of alkalosis), cerebral blood flow, blood pressure, and survival.
  ● *BVM:* Cricoid pressure, surgilube on face if poor seal
■ **DDx:** "ABCDE" (**A**ir, **B**lood, **C**atecholamines, **D**rugs, **E**lectrolytes). Clues: Meds, PMH, procedures
  ● *Exam:* JVD, track marks, lungs, shunt, pulse with CPR?
  ● *Tests:* Glu, Hb, K, ABG, CXR, echo
■ **LV Assist Device:** No compressions: unit has its own pump. Disconnect battery to shock. Use normal drugs
■ **Trauma:** Asystole = dead; no pulse = needs a thoracotomy and bilateral chest tubes
■ **Confirm:** Asystole: In two leads; PEA: Doppler, echo; VF: leads OK? VT: 12 lead, synchronize if pulse
■ **Intubation:** $ETCO_2$ (values < 5 mEq/l associated with very low probability of survival)
■ **Results:** If arrest in the hospital 18% survive to discharge. If arrest in community, < 10% go home.

TREATMENT
■ **1st ABCs:** Airway, breathing, CPR, defib x 1/thump
■ **2nd ABCs:** A: ETT, B: Confirm; C: IV, rhythm
■ **Countershocks:** Don't stack, gel, sync, dry off sweat, shave hair, O_2 off. Internal paddles: use 1/10th J.
■ **Pitfalls:** Forgetting to synch; forgetting to turn off O_2; forgetting to avoid pacer, nipples, and NTG
■ **ACLS 2005:** Recommends start at highest energies if pulseless; no rhythm/pulse check until 2 min CPR.

TABLE 7.1.   Initial Countershock Levels for Various Dysrhythmias

Phase Type	VF/VT s̄ pulse	VT c̄ Pulse	A-Fib	Flutter, SVT	Peds: VF/VT	Peds: Other
Monophasic	360 J	100 J	100 J	50 J	2 J/kg > 4 J/kg	1 J/k > 2J/k
Biphasic	120–200	75 J	50 J	10–25 J	2 J/kg > 4 J/kg	0.25 J/k–0.5 J/k

Source: Pregerson DB. *Quick Essentials Emergency Medicine 4.0.* ERPocketbooks.com; 2010:219.

■ **Pacing:** Rate = 80 (or slower in MI), current 20–200 mAmps (set at capture + 2mA), full-demand mode
  • *Capture:* Wide QRS, ST&T waves, pulse; get a 12 lead; ↑mAmps or ↑pulse with: CHF, COPD, fat
  • *Comps:* 3rd-degree burn (clip, don't shave hair), hiccups if too close to diaphragm
  • *Venous:* Attach V lead, look for injury current. Start at 5 mAmps, full-demand mode
  • *Post:* CXR, tip should be in apex of right ventricle

MEDICATION BASICS
■ **General:** IV running = flush, proximal IV. Make sure to kink when pushing IV infiltrating? Raise arm!
  • *ETT meds:* Endotracheal tube drugs use 2x dose: "NAVEL" (**N**arcan, **A**tropine, **V**alium, **E**pi, **L**idocaine). But if patient intubated, no need to give Narcan as risk > benefit once intubated.
  • *IO line:* Preferred over using ET tube for meds. See Section 3: Procedure (pages 69–100) for more information.
  • *Pitfalls:* Forgetting to start a drip after conversion; Adenosine without the crash cart

ASYSTOLE
■ **Prognosis:** Survival is about 1% for asystole
■ **DDx:** ↑: K, H+, tox. ↓: O_2, BP, temp, K, glucose. Clot: MI, PE. Obstructive: tamp, PTX, AutoPEEP
  • *Clues:* "PEACH" (**P**ulse with CPR? **E**KG/echo/FAST, **A**BG, **C**XR, **H**ard to bag?)
  • *Exam:* Cold? trauma? pupils? JVD? trachea? scar? lungs? shunt? tracks? DVT?
■ **Rx:** "FECES" (**F**luid (helps: bleed, shock, tamponade, PTX, OD, ↑K), **E**TT, **C**PR, **E**pi, **S**earch for a treatable Dx).
  • *Meds:* Epi 1 mg q3–5m, atropine 1 mg (max. 3 mg)
■ **Consider:** Atropine, bicarb, CaCl 10 ml IVP, dextrose, epi, fluid, glucagon 5 mg IVP, Narcan, tPA; but previous not for routine use. Without good reason, bicarb and calcium more likely to harm.

PEA
■ **Prognosis:** Survival is < 5% for PEA; worse if slow HR, wide QRS, no P-waves
■ **DDx:** ↑: K, H+, tox. ↓: O_2, BP, temp, K, glucose. Clot: MI, PE. Obstructive: tamp, PTX, AutoPEEP.
  • *Clues:* "PEACH" (**P**ulse with CPR? **E**KG/echo/FAST, **A**BG, **C**ardiac monitor, **C**XR, **H**ct, **H**ard to bag?)
  • *Exam:* Doppler; cold? trauma? pupils? JVD? trachea? scar? lungs? shunt? tracks? DVT?
■ **Rx:** "FECES" (**F**luid [good for: bleed, shock, tamponade, PTX, OD, ↑K], **E**TT, **C**PR, **E**pi, **S**earch for Rx'able Dx).
  • *Meds:* Epi 1mg q3–5m, atropine 1 mg for slow PEA (max. 3 mg)
■ **Consider:** Atropine, bicarb, CaCl 10 ml IVP, dextrose, epi, fluid, glucagon 5 mg IVP, Narcan, tPA; but previous not for routine use. Without good reason, bicarb and calcium more likely to harm.

PULSELESS V-TACH AND V-FIB
■ **DDx:** MI, LYTES (acid/K/Mg), DRUG (cocaine, TCA, heroin), cold, tamp/PTX, pacer-mediated
■ **Rx:** Shock x1 at max joules then CPR at 30:2 ratio without pulse check for 2 min before reshock. Pressors: epi 1mg IV q3–5m; drugs: Amiodarone 300 mg (may repeat at 150 mg) – equal recommendation to lidocaine; lidocaine 1.5 mg/kg (100 mg, may repeat half dose up to 3 mg/kg max) also first line. Torsades: defib; magnesium 2 g/2 min then 2–4 mg/min and overdrive pace or Isuprel to keep HR > 90
■ **Amio vs. Lido:** Admit: 23% vs. 12%; home: 5% vs. 3%; but groups different! ACLS does NOT recommend amio 1st

BRADYCARDIA
■ **DDx:** Low: O_2, glucose, temp. High: K, Trop, TSH. Tox: Amio., BB, CCB, Dig, clonidine, Li. Other: Sick Sinus Syndrome...
■ **Rx:** O_2, pace, atropine 0.5mg/dose (max 3 mg), dopamine at 2–10mcg/kg/m, epi at 2–10 mcg/m
  • *Other:* Calcium for ↑K, glucagon 1–5 mg for BB or CCB tox, Fab for Dig tox, (theophyline, Isuprel)
  • *Atropine:* Give 0.5mg first (Caution in MI and Mobitz 2nd or 3rd degree AVB because increases VT/VF)
■ **Mobitz I:** DDx: vagal, degenerative, ischemia, meds, Carditis (Chaga's, Lyme, diphtheria, etc.)
■ **Mobitz II:** DDx: degenerative, anterior MI, calcified aortic valve. Rx: Pacer
■ **3° AVB:** DDx: AMI, congenital, post-op, trauma, carditis, Ca↑ or ↓. Rx: Pacer

TACHYCARDIA: WIDE WITH A PULSE

■ **General:** If unstable, then cardiovert (synch first). Use ONE drug max. Assume V-tach

■ **Regular:** Amiodarone 150 mg/10 min + drip > sync and cardiovert. Adenosine can fix some VT (admit ICU)
   ● *V-Tach*: > 30 sec. = sustained VT; rate 120–200, often 3°AVB, QRS >140 and concordant, extreme LAD
   ● *DDx*: SVT with aberrancy, WPW, AIVR (rate usually < 120), hyperkalemia (rate usually < 120)

■ **Irregular**
   ● *A-fib and BBB*: Rx as A-fib
   ● *WPW and A-fib*: May look regular
   ● *Rx*: Cardiovert (Amio), Procainamide. NO: Adenosine, dig, CCB, BB. Amiodarone has properties of BB and CCB. Torsade: Rx: Cardiovert, fix electrolytes and ischemia, magnesium 1–2 g over 5–50 min.

TABLE 7.2.   Drugs for Wide Complex Tachydysrhythmias

Drug	Fix (%)	Side Effects	Dosing	Max
Lidocaine	20	Safest; seize if push fast	1.5 mg/kg IVP; repeat 0.75 mg/kg	3 mg/kg
Amiodaron	80	Low BP; long QT	300 mg IVP; repeat 150 mg	2.2 g/24 hr
Magnesium	40	Flushing; ↓BP (usually mild drop)	2 mg IVP	Monitor mg level

TACHYCARDIA: NARROW WITH A PULSE

■ **General:** If unstable, then cardiovert (synch 1st). Only use one drug after adenosine. All proarrhythmic.
   ● *Rates*: < 150: If unstable likely 2nd cause; > 150: may be unstable; > 200: more likely to be WPW
   ● *Rate control*: Use diltiazem or beta blockers (preferred in setting of ischemia; avoid if CHF or COPD/RAD).

■ **Irregular:** Always look for precipitant such as fever, pain, dehydration, electrolytes, etc.
   ● *DDx*: A-fib, A-flutter, MAT; can also be sinus tach with PACs which is treated as sinus tach
   ● *Rx*: Control rate with diltiazem or beta-blocker, (heparin), ASA. Cardioversion risks acute CVA, especially if > 48 hr. of arrhythmia

■ **Regular:** Vagal maneuvers (valsalva best), adenosine converts SVT but usually not others
   ● *DDx*: SVT (u converts with vagal maneuvers or adenosine), A-flutter, junctional-tachycardia, PAT
   ● *Rx*: Vagal > adenosine > if persists control rate with diltiazem or beta-blocker, treat underlying dz.
   ● *Adenosine*: For: Stable, narrow, rate < 200 (if > 200 consider WPW before trying adenosine)
   ● *Dose*: 6 mg > 12 mg > 12 mg, but 3 mg starting dose if on Aggrenox, Tegretol, or Persantine

INDUCED HYPOTHERMIA AND POST-ARREST CARE

■ **Background**: Used since 1950s in cardiac surgery to protect brain and heart. Hypothermia decreases energy use, oxygen consumption, metabolism, and neurotoxic mediators.

■ **Studies:** N = 77, 12h at 33C then actively rewarmed x 6h. NNT = 4. All received Versed + vecuronium to prevent shivering and lidocaine infusion to prevent VT. HACA Study Group: N = 275, 24h at 32–34C then passively rewarm. NNT = 6. (Bernard SA, Gray TW, Buist MD, et al. Treatment of comatose survivors of out-of-hospital cardiac arrest with induced hypothermia. *NEJM*. 2002:346;557–563.)

■ **Indication:** Medical arrest, regains pulse but cannot follow commands or GCS < 9, going to ICU. Benefit: Best data in V-tach and V-fib. Class IIa: NNT=6. Improved survival and neurologic outcome.

■ **Contras:** Hypotension despite pressors, recurrent VT/VF, pregnant, active bleeding, ischemic digits.

■ **Relative:** Hypoxemia, pregnant, hypotension, other cause of coma, bleeding diathesis, pregnant, sepsis.

■ **Induction:** Start within 5 minutes. Cooled IV fluids (4C) via rapid infuser can drop 1C/L, then blanket. Goal 32-34C. Rectal temp lags core temp so need esophageal probe until in steady state.

■ **Maintenance:** Cooling blanket, prevent shivering (benzos, narcotics, paralytics all okay short term). Can use bladder temp probe once induction complete. Keep at 32-34C for 12–24h.

■ **Comps:** Overcooling, dysrhythmia (brady, VF), pneumonia/sepsis, bleeding, slowed drug metabolism, electrolyte shifts (K, Ca), seizure.

■ **Cost:** Can be as cheap as $25/day.

OTHER POST-ARREST CARE

■ **Blood Pressure:** Post-arrest cardiac stunning often starts 20–30min after ROSC and may last 24–48h
   ● *Rx*: Fluids, pressors, dobutamine (milrinone may be needed if beta blocked)
   ● *Volume*: Passive leg raise preload test: If raise legs to 45° and BP rises in next minute, they need fluids
   ● *MAP push*: To get good brain perfusion aim for MAP (Mean Arterial Pressure) >80 or at least MAP >65
■ **Ventilation:** Aim for oxygen sat of 95%. Too high can be damaging and increase free radicals
   ● *Protective*: Keep volumes low. Avoid aspiration by elevating HOB 45°
■ **Dx Cause:** EKG, labs, RUSH ultrasound protocol to diagnose cause of shock.
   ● *STEMI*: Cath lab and tPA both OK post-arrest per ILCOR
■ **CNS:** Check GSC and brainstem reflexes (corneals, pupils, gag, overbreathing the vent)
■ **Organ Donor:** Call organ procurement

DEATH AND DEATH TELLING

■ **Death:** Consider a moment of silence or a short prayer for patient.Do not sign death certificate. It can lead to liability.
■ **Deathtelling:** Quiet place. Introduce self. Find out what they already know. Relate highlights of care. Make certain you clearly tell them their loved-one died, but do this last. Recommend they view the deceased to say goodbye. Be available to answer questions.
■ **Family:** Family presence during CPR: Decide on case by case basis.Brief first then enter with dedicated staff member to explain and escort out if they impede care.

SHOCK AND PRESSORS

PULMONARY EDEMA AND HYPOTENSION

■ **General:** Consider Foley, ABG, lactate, echo, CVP, Swan. Rx with O_2, consider 2 L IV fluids before PRBCs or pressors, treat arrhythmia

■ **SBP and Rx:** > 100: NTG. 70–100: dobutamine if no sx/sn of shock, o/w dopamine. < 70: norepinephrine

■ **Goals:** MAP is most important. Keep 65–75. Is patient symptomatic? (AMS, CP, weak)

■ **Positioning:** Trendelenberg: no good evidence and potential for harm (↓cardiac output, ↓tidal volume)

■ **Consider:** "SINC" (Steroids, IABP, Narcan, Calcium); also consider bicarb for OD, acidosis

■ **Pressors:** Data from small trials or animal studies; titrate to MAP of 65–70, not higher. No evidence that outcome improved. IV fluids and early Rx of primary cause most important. Use with caution in right-sided MI or cardiac valvular pathology.

TABLE 7.3. Types of Shock and Management

Shock Type	Causes	Treatment (DA = Dopamine, NE = Nor-Epi)	Tests
Hypovolemic	Hemorrhage	IVF, blood, surgery	Serial Hb
	Dehydration	IVF, check electrolytes	Chemistry
Obstructive	PE	Heparin > (tPA, NorEpinephrine [NE]) Careful IVF (bulging RV means less LV volume)	Echo CT, VQ
	TPTX, tamponade	Needle, drainage	XR, echo
Cardiogenic	CHF, MI, valve	SBP > 80: Dobutamine; SBP < 80: Dopamine SBP < 70: NE, IABP, repair	Echo, trop, Ca+
Distributive	Sepsis	ABX and IV fluid > (replete calcium) > (steroid) > NE + Dobutamine	Cultures, CBC, lactate
	Addison's	Steroids, D50, IVF	Cortisol
	Neurogenic	IV fluid, Dopamine (DA) > NE	CT, MR
	Tricyclic OD	Bicarb, NE + Dobutamine (not DA)	EKG
	Anaphylaxis	EPI, H1, H2, glucagon, IVF, steroid	H and P

Source: Pregerson DB. *Quick Essentials Emergency Medicine 4.0.* ERPocketbooks.com; 2010:52.

TABLE 7.4. Pressors Comparison

Pressor	Indication	Dosing	Alpha*	Beta1*	Beta2*	DA	If on BB
Dopamine	Cardiac, spine	2–20 μ/k/m	++	+++	++	++++	May fail
Dobutamine	Septic, CHF	2–20 μ/k/m	+	++++	++	0	May fail
Epinephrine	Anaphylaxis	1–4 (-10) μ/m	+++	++++	+++	0	May fail
Glucagon	Allergic, OD	1–5 mg	0	0	0	0	Works
Milrinone	CHF	50 μ/k + drip	0	0	0	0	Works
Norepinephrine**	Sepsis, CHF	20 (30) μ/m	++++	++++	+	0	May fail
Phenylephrine**	Shock, on BB	20–200 μ/m	++++	0	0	0	Works
Vasopressin	Sepsis: 2nd drug	2.4 unit/hr	0	0	0	0	Works

* Adverse Effectis: Alpha: gangrene; Beta1: arrhythmia, MVO₂; Beta2: hypotension
** Best Choices: Levophed = Norepinephrine; Neo-Synephrine = Phenylephrine cause less dysrhythmia and may decrease mortality
Source: Pregerson DB. *Quick Essentials Emergency Medicine 4.0.* ERPocketbooks.com; 2010:51.

TABLE 7.5. Non-Pressor Agents That May Raise Blood Pressure

Others	Indications	Dosing	Notes
Bicarbonate	TCA OD, ↓pH	1–4 amp + drip	Causes hypokalemia, hypernatremia, shift O_2 curve
Calcium*	↑K+, ↓Ca++	1–3 amp + drip	CaCl immediate onset; Ca-gluc: 30-min delay onset
Decadron	Addisonian	6–10 mg IV	Send Cortisol level; can suppress immune system

*Calcium: 3 amps gluconate = 1 amp CaCl. Calcium is a potential cellular toxin.
Source: Pregerson DB. *Quick Essentials Emergency Medicine 4.0.* ERPocketbooks.com; 2010:51.

HIGHLIGHTS OF CRITICAL CARE DRUGS

General: In cardiac arrest flush with 20 ml, then elevate arm for 20 sec. during CPR. The following drugs cause hypokalemic arrhythmias: Lasix, epinephrine, bicarb, albuterol. All drugs have the potential to worsen outcome, even in a pulseless patient. Correct electrolyte abnormalities first if possible.

Medics: ETT dose: Atropine 1 mg, lidocaine 3 mg/kg; NTG in CHF 0.8 mg, if SBP > 150 may repeat.

■ **ACE Inhibitor**: For AMI, CHF, HTN. Dose: Enalaprilat 0.625–1.25 mg IV.
  ● *Cautions*: Pregnancy, creatinine > 2 (> 2.5 for men), renal artery stenosis, K > 5, low BP

■ **Adenosine**: For PSVT. Dose: 6 mg (3 mg if on persantine, Aggrenox, or tegretol) >12mg > 12mg.
  ● *Cautions*: Poisoning, heart block, WPW + A-fib.

■ **Amiodarone**: For VT, VF, AF. Dose: VF: 300 mg IVP. Alt.: 150 mg/10 min + drip.
  ● *Cautions*: Long QT (WPW), side effects (long QT, low BP, thyroid, bradycardia), interacts.

■ **Atropine**: For symptomatic brady, asystole/PEA, OD. Dose: 0.5–1 mg (max. 3 mg except some ODs).
  ● *Cautions*: MI (increases O_2 demand), hypothermia, won't work if infranodal.

■ **Bicarb**: For hyperkalemia, certain ODs, long arrest. Dose: 1 mEq/kg.
  ● *Cautions*: Hypokalemia, not for routine use; good CPR and ventilation far more important.

■ **Calcium**: For hyperkalemia, hypocalcemia, some ODs. Dose: CaCl more rapid effect: 1 amp.
  ● *Cautions*: Not for routine cardiac arrest; calcium gluconate may take 30 min before effect.

■ **Digibind**: For severe digoxin OD (and K > 5, dig. level > 10). Dose: 3–10 vials.
  ● *Cautions*: Measured digoxin levels rise after use and so are unreliable.

■ **Diltiazem**: For rate control in A-fib or A-flutter. Dose: 10–20 mg boluses, drip at 5–15 mg/h.
  ● *Cautions*: Poisonings, wide complex tachycardia, WPW and A-fib, concurrent beta blocker.

■ **Dobutamine**: For CHF with SBP 70–100 and no signs of shock. Dose: 2–20 mcg/kg/min.
  ● *Cautions*: Poisoning, shock.

■ **Dopamine**: For bradycardia, SBP 70–100 and signs of shock. Dose: 2–20 mcg/kg/min.
  ● *Cautions*: Correct hypovolemia before use, causes tachycardia and vasoconstriction.

■ **Epinephrine**: For VF, VT, asystole, PEA, bradycardia, anaphylaxis. Dose: 1 mg IV q3–5 min. Drip: 2–20 mcg/min.
  ● *Cautions*: Hypokalemia, "high-dose" epi leads to worse outcome except in poisonings, etc.

■ **Esmolol**: For aortic dissection, HTN emergency. Dose: 500 mcgs/kg bolus + 50 mcg/kg/min.
  ● *Cautions*: Asthma, bradycardia, cocaine, CHF, concurrent verapamil or diltiazem.

■ **Glucagon**: For beta blocker or calcium blocker toxicity, anaphylaxis if on beta blocker. Dose: 3 mg, then 3 mg/h.
  ● *Cautions*: Vomiting, hyperglycemia.

■ **Inamrinone**: For severe CHF refractory to other agents. Dose: 0.75 mg/kg over 10 min and 5–1 5mcg/k/m.
  ● *Cautions*: Tachycardia, low BP, myocardial ischemia.

■ **Lidocaine**: For VF, VT. Less toxic/cheaper than amio. Onset 1 min. Dose: 1–1.5 mg/kg then 1–4 mg/min.
  ● *Cautions*: Prophylactic use in AMI, use half dose in perfusing rhythm, max. dose is 3 mg/kg.

■ **Magnesium**: For Torsade, low magnesium suspected, dig. toxicity. Dose: 1–2 g over 5–60 min.
  ● *Cautions*: Renal failure, prophylactic use, drop in BP possible.

■ **Metoprolol**: For ACS, aortic dissection. Dose: 5 mg IV x 3 prn.
  ● *Cautions*: Asthma, bradycardia, cocaine, CHF, concurrent verapamil or diltiazem.

■ **Nitroprusside**: For aortic dissection, hypertensive emergency. Dose: titrate to pain and vitals.
  ● *Cautions*: This is more an afterload reducer than is NTG and is more rapidly titratable.

■ **Nor-Epi**: For shock, especially if septic, cardiogenic, neurogenic or TCA overdose. Dose: 2–8–30 mcg/min.
  ● *Cautions*: Correct hypovolemia before use, causes tachycardia and vasoconstriction

■ **NTG**: For ischemic chest pain, CHF. Dose: start 10 mg/min., titrate to pain and vitals.
  ● *Cautions*: SBP < 90–105, pulse < 60 or > 100, inferior MI, RV-MI, Viagra/Cialis/Levitra.

■ **PGE1**: For congenital cyanotic heart disease. Dose: 0.05–0.1 mcg/kg, then titrate up.
  ● *Cautions*: Sides: Apnea, fever, agitation, seizures, hypoglycemia, hypocalcemia, low BP.

■ **Pronestyl**: For stable VT and normal QT, PSVT, WPW with A-fib. Onset up to 10 min. Dose: 20–50 mg/min IV, max: 17 mg kg. Drip 1–6 mg/min (lower in CHF, L, RI).
  ● *Cautions*: Prolongs QT, lowers BP, contraindicated in MG, onset up to 10 min.

■ **Vasopressin**: For alternative to epi for VF, asystole, PEA. Dose: 40 units once.
  ● *Cautions*: Can cause extravasation necrosis.

BASICS
Usually hypoxic, airway or septic arrest rather than primary cardiac.
- **Red Flags:** RR > 60 or grunting/retractions, HR <80 or > 180 or poor perfusion, AMS, Sz, trauma, sepsis
- **Formulae:** Kg = 10 + 2(age in years) For age < 1y: 4 + (age in months/2)
  - *Vitals:* Normal BP = 90 + (age)(2). Low normal BP = 70 + (age)(2). Normal max HR <180 - 10(age)
- **Shock DDx:** "THE MIST" (**T**rauma, **H**eart (No CCB age <1), **E**ndocrine, **M**etabolic, **I**ntestine, **S**epsis, **T**ox)
- **CPR:** Ratios: 1 rescuer - 30:2. 2 rescuers - 15:2. Thumb CPR best age<1, RR = 20, HR = 100. Give 2 minutes CPR (5 cycles) after defibrillation and BEFORE rhythm/pulse check. Start CPR for HR <60 and poor perfusion even if there is a pulse
- **Electricity:** As long as paddles one inch apart they're OK. Start 2 J/kg if pulseless, 0.5–1 J/kg if pulse
- **Glucose:** Check it, it's often low. D25: 2–4 ml/kg, but if age <3 mo use D10: 5–10 ml/kg
- **Lines:** 4 French. Controversial if femoral of subclavian best. Try EJ first.
  - *IV:* Push bolus via syringe rather than using a line
  - *IO:* 5 ml flush after meds. Proximal tibia or distal femur
- **Tubes:** ET Tubes: 4 + years/4 and round down. Use 1 size smaller for cuffed ET tubes. Chest Tube: 4 x ETT. NG and Foley: 2 x ETT, 12 French

AIRWAY
- **Death:** Airway and drowning > SIDS > respiratory > MVA > fire, suffocation, poison
- **Choking:** If complete obstruction: Age >1: Heimlich. Age<1: 5 back blows and 5 chest thrusts. No blind finger sweeps (may push FB deeper)
- **ET Tubes:** Cuffed tube preferred: size = 3 + years/4. In neonates use uncuffed: size = 3–4
- **Blades:** Preterm: Miller 0 Term: Miller 1 1y: Miller 1 2y: Miller 2 12y: Mac 3
- **Atropine:** Use to premedicate age <5 (and in adults who get succ repeated or start bradycardic):

PULSELESS ARREST
Outcomes poor, prevent arrest by early intervention
- **Asystole/PEA:** CPR, fluids, ETT, search for cause, epinephrine 0.01 mg/kg IV/IO q3–5 min, pace. atropine not in peds pulseless arrest algorithm, but may consider. Min. dose 0.1 mg
- **VF/VT:** Shock 2 J/kg, then 4 J/kg, CPR, epinephrine 0.01 mg/kg IV/IO q3–5min.
  - *Drugs:* Lidocaine 1 mg/kg + drip at 20–50 mcg/min, amiodarone 5 mg/kg, magnesium 25–50 mg/kg

ARRYTHMIAS AND SHOCK
- **Bradycardia:** Preterminal rhythm: O_2 by BVM > CPR if HR< 60 when poor perfusion even if has a pulse. > epi 0.01 mg kg > atropine 0.02/kg (min. dose 0.1 mg, max. total 1 mg) > pace
- **Tachycardia:** Sinus, SVT or wide? SVT rate usually > 220 in infant and 180 in peds
  - *Wide:* Rx: 0.5–1 J/kg > 2 J/kg > amiodarone 5 mg/kg over 20–60' or Procainamide 15 mg/kg over 30–60' or lidocaine 1 mg/kg IV bolus (only one you can bolus)
  - *Narrow:* SVT Rx: Vagal (ice bag/rag to face, make them cry) > adenosine 0.1 mg/kg > 0.5–1 J/kg > amio. NO calcium blockers age < 1 yr.
- **Septic:** Give fluid boluses of 20 ml/kg x three or more depending on response. Early ABX. Correct low calcium and low glucose. If BP remains low, consider solu-cortef 2 mg/kg and pressors.
  - *Pressors:* Norepi at 0.1–2 mcg/kg/m if "warm" shock, epi if "cold" shock.
- **Trauma:** Consider blood (10 ml/kg PRBCs) after 2nd or 3rd fluid bolus of 20 ml/kg (sooner if severe).
- **PGE1:** Ductal dependent lesion: dose: 0.05–0.1 mcg/k/m (Sides: ↓BP, apnea, fever, Sz, ↓glucose/Ca).

TABLE 7.6.   Pediatric and Neonatal Critical Care Drug Dosing

Dose	Pediatric Drugs for that Dose	Dose	Drugs
0.01 mg/k	Epinephrine, Flumazenil	0.02 mg/kg	Atropine: min dose 0.1 mg
0.1 mg/k	Narcan, Benzos, Adenosine, Decadron (0.15/k)	0.3 mg/kg	Etomidate
1 mg/k	Roc, lido, bicarb (mEq), Benadryl, Prednisone	2 mg/kg	Succ, Gent, Solucortef
5 mg/kg	Amiodarone		
10 mg/k	Vanco (15/k), EES; Dilantin and Phenobarb (MRx1)	50 mg/kg	Beta-lactams, magnesium
1 g/k	Kayexylate, charcoal	2 ml/kg	D25 (D10 5 ml/kg if < 3 mon)

- *Dextrose*: Neonate: D10 at 5–10 ml/kg; age > 1: D25: 2 ml/kg. Shortcut: D5NS 20ml/kg bolus, may repeat x1
- *Drips*: Epi 0.1–1 mcg/kg/min, Norepi 0.1–2 mcg/kg/min

■ THE BROSELOW TAPE

- *Accuracy*: Within 10% in only 60% of kids; underestimates weight/dosing more often
- *Obesity*: Big reason for underestimating. More important for lipophilic drugs (i.e., Versed, amiodarone)

NEONATAL RESUSCITATION

- **General:** Neonate = 0–3 mon. Response = ↑HR (umbilical pulse). Kg = 4 + months/2
- **Vitals:** Normal: HR: 100–180, RR: 30–60, BP: 55/26–90/55. Consider OG tube as gas in stomach > poor ventilation and aspiration risk.
- **Meconium:** Low HR, RR, or tone: Don't stimulate, De Lee suction followed by endotracheal suctioning. If vigorous: No suction even if thick
- **1st 30 Seconds:** "DWSP" (**D**ry, **W**arm, **S**timulate, **P**osition); suction: mouth > nose, then OK to stimulate
- **2nd 30 Seconds:** If cyanotic, give supplemental O_2, if apneic or HR < 100, give by BVM at 40–60
- **3rd 30 Seconds:** If HR < 60 or < 80 and not ↑ing, perform CPR (90 compressions and 30 breaths/min, ratio 3:1)
  - ↑ HR (umbilical pulse) is best indicator of improvement
- **4th 30 Seconds:** If HR still < 60, administer drugs: epi > Narcan 0.1 mg/k > D10 and consider IV fluids
- **Tubes:** ET tube: Weeks/size: 25 wks/2.5, 30 wks/3.0, > 35 wks/3.5
- **Lines:** Umbilical line = 4 French: Advance 4 cm
- **Survival:** Intact survival: 22 wks or < 500g: 0%; 23 wks or 500–600 g: 30%; 24 wks or 600–700 g: 60%; 25 wks or 700–800 g: 70%; 26 wks or 800–900 g: 80%; 28 wks or 900–1000g: 90%

TABLE 7.7. APGAR Scores

Heart Rate	0: none	1 point: < 100	2 points: >100
Resp. Rate	0: none	1 point: slow	2 points: good
Tone	0: limp	1 point: fair	2 points: active motion
Irritability	0: none	1 point: grimace	2 points: cough, cry
Color	0: blue/pale	1 point: blue arms/legs	2 points: pink all over

APPENDICES

COMMON MEDICAL TERMS TRANSLATED

ARABIC (ARABI)			
NUMBERS		Diabetes	Sukari
one, two	wahed, itnen	Disease	Amrad
three, four	thabata, arba	Dizzy	Dayekh
five, six	hamsa, setta	Doctor	Tabeeb
A		Drink	Ishrab
Abdomen	Albaten	**E**	
Alcohol	Kuhul	Ear	Uthun
Allergy	Hassasiyeh	Eat	Kul
A little	Kalil	Elbow	Cou'
A lot	Katheer	Eye	Ayen
Angiogram	Takhteet	**F**	
Anxiety	Mutareeb	Fever	Harrara
Appendix	Al-Zaeida	Finger	Isba'a
Appetite	Shaheeh	Foot	Kadam
Arm	Theraa	**G**	
Artery	Shirian	Gallbladder	Marara
Arthritis	Romatism	Go	Hena
B		Good	Gayed
Back	Khallef	**H**	
Bad	Saaeh	Hand	Yaed
Better	Ahsan	Hard/heavy	Gamed
Big	Kabeer	Have	Aindy
Blood	Daem	Head	Raas
Brain	Akel	Headache	Sudaa
Breathe	Nafas	Heart	Kaleb
Breathing	Tanafess	Help	Khadmeh
Burns	Huruk	Here	Huna
C		Home	Manzel
Cancer	Cancer	Hospital	Mustashfa
Chest	Sader	Hours	Sa'at
Cough	Kuhaa	How long	Kam al zaman
D		How many	Kadaish
Days	Ayam	HTN	Daghet
Defecation	Yataraz		

I

I, me	Ana
Injection	Hukna
Intestines	Amaa

K

Kidneys	Kalawee
Knee	Rukbeh

L

Lab tests	Fahes Mukhtabar
Last	Akheer
Leg	Regel
Liver	Kabed
LOC or KO	Fukdan Wayee
Lungs	Ria'a

M

Medicine	Elag
Muscle	Adalat

N

Nausea	Dyekheh
Nerve	Asaab
No	La
Now	Alaan
Nurse	Mumareeda

P

Pain	Wagaa
Please	Lau Samaht
Pneumonia	Pneumonia
Pressure	Daghet

S

Same	Mesle
Sharp (pain)	Ha'ad
Short breath	Deek Nafas
Shoulder	Katef
Sick	Mareed
Small	Sageer
Sorry	Assef
Spine	Amoud Fakari
Sputum	Mokat

Start	Intalek
Stomach	Maeedeh
Stool	Fadalat
Stop	Kuff
Stroke	Faleg
Strong	Kawee
Surgery	Amleyeh
Sweat	Tareek
Swollen	Waram

T

Tetanus	Tetanus
This	Hatha
Throat	Hungaraa/Zoor
Thyroid	Al Gudeh Al Dorakey
Transfusion	Tahweel
Tuberculosis	Tuberculosis

U

Ulcer	Kurha
Urine	Pawel

V

Valve	Samam
Vein	Al Areek
Vomiting	Yurageh

W

Want	Aureed
Weak	Daeefl
Weakness	Daeef
What	Matha
When	Mata
Where	Ayen
Who	Man
Worse	Aswaa

X

X-ray	Asheaa

Y

Yes	Naem
You	Anta
Your	Laak

ARMENIAN (HAYEREN)

NUMBERS

one, two	meg, yergoo
three, four	yerek, tchors
five, six	hink, vets

A

Abdomen	Por
Alcohol	Alcogol
Allergy	Alergia
A little	Pokr
A lot	Shat
Angiogram	Anjiograma
Anxiety	Agrvats
Appendix	Kuiraghik
Appetite	Ahurdjak
Arm	Dzerk
Artery	Yerak
Arthritis	Hotat tsav

B

Back	Meshk
Bad	Vut
Better	Avelilav
Big	Mets
Blood	Arune
Brain	Ughegh
Breathe	Shunch
Breathing	Shunchel
Burns	Airvatskner

C

Cancer	Kahtskeh
Chest	Kurtskivantag
Cough	Haz

D

Days	Ayam
Defecation	Gherdel
Diabetes	Shakarahd
Disease	Hivantutyoon
Dizzy	Glhaptuit
Doctor	Bjishk
Drink	Hmel

E

Ear	Akange
Eat	Ker
Elbow	Armug
Eye	Achk

F

Fever	Takutyoon
Finger	Mut
Foot	Votk

G

Gallbladder	Lehapark
Go	Kna
Good	Lav

H

Hand	Tat
Hard/heavy	Ujeh/tsanrutsun
Have	Uni
Head	Gluhe
Headache	Glhatsav
Heart	Seart
Help	Oknutsun
Here	Hos
Home	Tun
Hospital	Hivantanots
Hours	Jamer
How long	Vorkan yergain
How many	Kani had
HTN	Djenshoom

I

I, me	Yes
Injection	Nermoodzel
Intestines	Ahikner

K

Kidneys	Yerikam
Knee	Tsunke

L

Lab tests	Airian kennutyun
Last	Verchi
Leg	Votk
Liver	Leyart
LOC or KO	Ushagnatsutsun
Lungs	Tocker

M

Medicine	Begh
Muscle	Mkan

N

Nausea	Sirtaharnots
Nerve	Cheegh
No	Che/voch
Now	Hima
Nurse	Bujkuir

P

Pain	Tsav
Please	Hintrem
Pneumonia	Tokaborb
Pressure	Chanshum
Pus	Tarakh

S

Same	Nooyn
Sharp (pain)	Tsakum tsav
Short breath	Shunchaktor
Shoulder	Us
Sick	Hivand
Small	Pokr
Sorry	Keneres
Spine	Vohnashar
Sputum	Horh
Start	Skisir
Stomach	Stamoks
Stool	Kahkank
Stop	Kahkni
Stroke	Katvats
Strong	Ujeh
Surgery	Virahatutyun

T

Sweat	Kahtsir
Swollen	Urats

T

Tetanus	Paitatsmandem sriskum
This	Ice
Throat	Cocort
Thyroid	Cocorti gehts
Transfusion	Iruny popohume
Tuberculosis	Tukaht

U

Ulcer	Hots
Urine	Mez

V

Valve	Yerak/klapan
Vein	Yerak
Vomiting	Peskhel

W

Want	Uzenal, uzel
Weak	Tule, degar
Weakness	Tulutyun
What	Inch
When	Yerp
Where	Wordeh, oor
Who	Ov
Worse	Vatanal

X

X-ray	Rentgen

Y

Yes	Ayo
You	Du
Your	Dzer/kon

NUMBERS

one, two	yi, ar
three, four	sen, seu
five, six	oo, liu

A

Abdomen	Du Ze
Alcohol	Geo
Allergy	Ming Gaan
A little	Yi Dian
A lot	Hen Duo
Angiogram	Sing Dao Guan
Anxiety	Jing Zhang
Appendix	Maan Chaan
Appetite	Wueh Koh
Arm	Sho
Artery	Shea Guan
Arthritis	Gwan jye yen

B

Back	Bei
Bad	Huai
Better	Gern How
Big	Da
Blood	Shea
Brain	Nao
Breathe	Hu Shi
Breathing	Hu Shi
Burns	Shao Saan

C

Cancer	Ai Jen
Chest	Xiong
Cough	Ke So

D

Days	Tian
Defecation	Da bian
Diabetes	Tan Niao Biin
Disease	Biin
Dizzy	Toe Huen
Doctor	Yi Seng
Drink	Herr

E

Ear	Earl
Eat	Chi
Elbow	Zhou
Eye	Yen Ging

F

Fever	Faa Shao
Finger	So Ze
Foot	Giao

G

Gallbladder	Daan
Go	Chu
Good	Hao

H

Hand	So
Hard/heavy	Zhung
Have	Yeo
Head	Toe
Headache	Toe Tong
Heart	Sing
Help	Bun Maan
Here	Tzeu li
Home	Tia
Hospital	Yee yuen
Hours	Shao sheu
How long	Do chi ohn
How many	Duo shao
HTN	Gao xe ya

I

I, me	Wo
Injection	Da jen
Intestines	Siao Chaan

K

Kidneys	Sheng Jang
Knee	Xi

L

Lab tests	Shea Hua Yen
Last	Jueh Ho
Leg	Giao

Liver	Gan
LOC or KO	Huen Dao
Lungs	Fei

M

Medicine	Yao
Muscle	Gi Lo

N

Nausea	Sian Tu
Nerve	Sen Ging
No	Boo
Now	Sian Jai
Nurse	Hu Se

P

Pain	Tun
Please	Ching
Pneumonia	Fei Ian
Pressure	Ya Li
Pus	Noone

S

Same	Yi yong
Sharp (pain)	Gian
Short breath	Hu Si Quen Naan
Shoulder	Gian
Sick	Biin
Small	Shiao
Sorry	Due bu chi
Spine	Bei Gi Gu
Sputum	Taan
Start	Kai Se
Stomach	Wei
Stool	Da Bian
Stop	Ting
Stroke	Zun Fong

Strong	Chiang
Surgery	Kai Dao
Sweat	Chu Hang
Swollen	Jun Da

T

Tetanus	Poor Sang Fung
This	Che ge
Throat	Ho Lun
Thyroid	Gia Zuan Siang
Transfusion	Su Shea
Tuberculosis	Fei Gie Ke

U

Ulcer	Hui Yang
Urine	Niao

V

Valve	Valvula
Vein	Jing Mai
Vomiting	Tu

W

Want	Yao
Weak	Ruo
Weakness	Ruo
What	Ahe mo
When	Gi Se
Where	Na Li
Who	Sui
Worse	Erhua

X

X-ray	X-guang

Y

Yes	Se
You	Ni
Your	Ni Te

FRENCH (FRANCAIS)

NUMBERS

one, two	un, dues
three, four	trois, quatre
five, six	cinq, six

A

Abdomen	Ventre
Alcohol	Alcool
Allergy	Allergie
A little	Peu de
A lot	Beaucoup
Angiogram	Angiogram
Anxiety	Anxiete
Appendix	Appendice
Appetite	Appetit
Arm	Bras
Artery	Artere
Arthritis	Arthrite

B

Back	Dos
Bad	Mal
Better	Meilleur
Big	Grand
Blood	Sang
Brain	Cerveau
Breathe	Respirer
Breathing	Respiration
Burns	Bruler

C

Cancer	Cancer
Chest	Poitrine
Cough	Tousser

D

Days	Jours
Defecation	Defecation
Diabetes	Diabetes
Disease	Maladie
Dizzy	Ne sens pa bien
Doctor	Docteur
Drink	Boire

E

Ear	Oreille
Eat	Manger
Elbow	Coude
Eye	Oeil

F

Fever	Fievre
Finger	Doigt
Foot	Pied

G

Gallbladder	Vesicule Biliaire
Go	Vont, Allez
Good	Bon, Bien

H

Hand	Main
Hard/heavy	Lourd
Have	Avoir
Head	Tete
Headache	Mal a la tete
Heart	Coeur
Help	Aider, Aide
Here	Ici
Home	Maison
Hospital	Hopital
Hours	Heures
How long	Combien du temps
How many	Combien
HTN	Hypertension

I

I, me	Je, Mois
Injection	L'injection
Intestines	Intestins

K

Kidney	Rein
Knee	Genou

L

Lab tests	Analyse du sang
Last	Dernier
Leg	Jambe

Liver	Foie
LOC or KO	Perte de conscience
Lungs	Poumons

M

Medicine	Medicine
Muscle	Muscle

N

Nausea	Nausea
Nerve	Nerf
No	Non
Now	Maintenant
Nurse	Infirmiere

P

Pain	Doleur
Please	S'il vous plait
Pneumonia	Pneumonie
Pressure	Pression
Pus	Pus

S

Same	Le meme
Sharp (pain)	Percant
Short breath	Je manque d'air
Shoulder	Epaule
Sick	Malade
Small	Petite
Sorry	Je sui desole
Spine	Epine
Sputum	Glaire
Start	Commencer
Stomach	Estomac
Stool	Selles
Stop	Areter
Stroke	Apoplexie

Strong	Forte
Surgery	Chirurgie
Sweat	Transpirer
Swollen	Tarabiscote'

T

Tetanus	Tetan
This	Ceci
Throat	Gorge
Thyroid	Thyroide
Transfusion	Transfusion
Tuberculosis	Tubercolosis

U

Ulcer	Ulcere
Urine	Urine

V

Valve	Abattant
Vein	Veine
Vomiting	Vomir

W

Want	Voudrais
Weak	Faible
Weakness	Faibilite
What	Quoi
When	Quand
Where	Ou
Who	Qui
Worse	Pire

X

X-ray	Radiographie

Y

Yes	Oui
You	Vous, Tu
Your	Votre, Ton

GERMAN (DEUTSCH)

NUMBERS

one, two	einz, zwei,
three, four	drei, vier
five, six	fuenf, sechs

A

Abdomen	Bauch
Alcohol	Alkohol
Allergy	Allergie
A little	Ein bisschen
A lot	Sehr
Angiogram	Angiogram
Anxiety	Angstzustand
Appendix	Blinddarm
Appetite	Appetit
Arm	Arm
Artery	Arterie
Arthritis	Rheuma

B

Back	Ruecken
Bad	Schlecht
Better	Besser
Big	Gross
Blood	Blut
Brain	Gehirn
Breathe	Atmen
Breathing	Atmung
Burns	Brandwunde

C

Cancer	Krebs
Chest	Brustkorb
Cough	Husten

D

Days	Tage
Defecation	Aufs Klo gehen
Diabetes	Diabetes
Disease	Krankheit
Dizzy	Schwindlig
Doctor	Arzt/Doktor
Drink	Trinken

E

Ear	Ohr
Eat	Essen
Elbow	Ellbogen
Eye	Auge

F

Fever	Fieber
Finger	Finger
Foot	Fuss

G

Gallbladder	Gallenblase
Go	Geh
Good	Gut

H

Hand	Hand
Hard/heavy	Schwer
Have	Haben
Head	Kopf
Headache	Kopfweh
Heart	Herz
Help	Hilfe
Here	Hier
Home	Zu Hause
Hospital	Krankenhaus
Hours	Stunden
How long	Wie lange
How many	Wie viele
HTN	Hoher Blut Druck

I

I, me	Ich
Injection	Injektion
Intestines	Darm

K

Kidneys	Nieren
Knee	Knie

L

Lab tests	Labortests
Last	Letzte/r
Leg	Bein
Liver	Leber

LOC or KO	Bewusstlosigkeit	Surgery	Operation
Lungs	Lungen	Sweat	Schweiss
		Swollen	geschwollen

M

Medicine	Medizin	**T**	
Muscle	Muskel	Tetanus	Tetanus

N

		This	Dieses
Nausea	Uebelkeit	Throat	Hals
Nerve	Nerv	Thyroid	Schilddruese
No	Nein	Transfusion	Transfusion
Now	Jetzt	Tuberculosis	Tuberkulose
Nurse	Krankenschwester		

P

		U	
		Ulcer	Magengeschwuer
Pain	Schmerz	Urine	Urin
Please	Bitte		
Pneumonia	Lungenentzuendung	**V**	
Pressure	Druck	Valve	Herzklappe
Pus	Eiter	Vein	Vene
		Vomiting	Erbrechen

S

		W	
Same	Gleich	Want	Wollen
Sharp (pain)	Stechend	Weak	Schwach
Short breath	Kurzatmigkeit	Weakness	Schwaeche
Shoulder	Schulter	What	Was
Sick	Krank	When	Wann
Small	Klein	Where	Wo
Sorry	Entschuldigung	Who	Wer
Spine	Wirbelsaeule	Worse	Schlimmer
Sputum	Schleim		
Start	Anfangen	**X**	
Stomach	Magen	X-ray	Roentgen
Stool	Stuhl/Kot		
Stop	Aufhoeren	**Y**	
Stroke	Schlaganfall	Yes	Ja
Strong	Stark	You	Sie
		Your	Ihr/Ihre

HEBREW (EEVREET)

NUMBERS

one, two	echad, shtiem
three, four	shalos, arba
five, six	hamesh, shesh

A

Abdomen	Beten
Alcohol	Alcohol
Allergy	Allergia
A little	Me'at
A lot	Harbe
Angiogram	Angiogram
Anxiety	Harada
Appendix	Toseftan
Appetite	Teavon
Arm	Zro'a
Artery	Oreq
Arthritis	Daleket prakim

B

Back	Gav
Bad	Ra
Better	Tov Yoter
Big	Gadol
Blood	Dam
Brain	Moah
Breathe	Linshom
Breathing	Respiracion
Burns	Kviot

C

Cancer	Sartan
Chest	Haze
Cough	Le-hishtael

D

Days	Yamim
Defecation	Hafrashat keyva
Diabetes	Suceret
Disease	Mahala
Dizzy	Seharhoreth
Doctor	Rofe
Drink	Lishthoth

E

Ear	Ozen
Eat	Le-ekhol
Elbow	Marpek
Eye	'Ayin

F

Fever	'Hom
Finger	Atsba
Foot	Regel

G

Gallbladder	Kis-Mara
Go	lech
Good	Tov

H

Have	Yesh
Head	Rosh
Headache	Keev Rosh
Heart	Lev
Help	Ezra
Here	Poe
Home	Habyit
Hospital	Beit cholim
Hours	Shaot
How long	Kama zman
How many	Kama
HTN	Lachatz dam gavoha

I

I, me	Anee
Injection	Ha zraka
Intestines	Me'aayim

K

Kidneys	Klayoth
Knee	Berekh

L

Lab tests	Bdikat M'aabada
Last	Akharon
Leg	Regel
Liver	Kaved
LOC or KO	Iboud Hakara
Lungs	Reot

M

Medicine	Refua
Muscle	Shrir

N

Nausea	Behila
Nerve	Atsav
No	Lo
Now	Akhshav
Nurse	Akhoth

P

Pain	Ke'ev
Please	Bevakasha
Pneumonia	Daleket Reot
Pressure	Lahats
Pus	Mugla

S

Same	Oto hadavar
Sharp (pain)	Had
Short breath	Katsar Neshima
Shoulder	Katef
Sick	Hole
Small	Kattan
Sorry	Mitztaair
Spine	Amud Shidra
Sputum	Kiyakh
Start	Hatkhel
Stomach	Keyva
Stool	Tsoah
Stop	Atsor
Stroke	Erua Mohi
Strong	Hazak
Surgery	Nituakh

Sweat	Lehazia
Swollen	Nafuach

T

Tetanus	Tetanus
This	Ze
Throat	Garon
Thyroid	Balutath Hamagen
Transfusion	Iruy Dam
Tuberculosis	Shahefeth

U

Ulcer	Kiv
Urine	Sheten

V

Valve	Mastem
Vein	Vrid
Vomiting	Meki

W

Want	Rotse
Weak	Halash
Weakness	Hulsha
What	Ma
When	Matai
Where	Efo
Who	Mi
Worse	Ra Yoter

X

X-ray	X-ray

Y

Yes	Ken
You	Ata
Your	Shelkha

INDONESIAN (BAHASA INDONESIA)

NUMBERS

one, two	satu, dua
three, four	tiga, empat
five, six	lima, enam

A

Abdomen	Abdomen
Alcohol	Alkohol
Allergy	Allergi
A little	Sedikit
A lot	Banyak
Angiogram	Angiogram
Anxiety	Nerves
Appendix	Usus Besar
Appetite	Nafsu makan
Arm	Lengan
Artery	Arteri
Arthritis	Artritis

B

Back	Belakang
Bed	Tempat tidur
Better	Lebih baik
Big	Besar
Blood	Darah
Brain	Otak
Breathe	Nafas
Breathing	Bernafas
Burns	Bakar

C

Cancer	Kanker
Chest	Dada
Cough	Batuk

D

Days	Hari
Defecation	Buang air besar
Diabetes	Diabetes
Disease	Penyakit
Dizzy	Pusing
Doctor	Doktor
Drink	Minum

E

Ear	Kuping/Telinga
Eat	Makan
Elbow	Sikut
Eye	Mata

F

Fever	Demam
Finger	Jari
Foot	Kaki

G

Gallbladder	Kantung
Go	Pergi
Good	Bagus

H

Hand	Tangan
Hard/heavy	Berat
Have	Punya
Head	Kepala
Headache	Sakit Kepala
Heart	Jantung
Help	Tolong
Here	Disini
Home	Rumah
Hospital	Rumah Sakit
Hours	Jam
How long	Berapa Lama
How many	Berapa Banyak
HTN	Tekanan dara tingi

I

I, me	Saya, saya
Injection	Suntik
Intestines	Usus

K

Kidneys	Ginjal
Knee	Lutut

L

Lab tests	Tes Lab
Last	Terakhir
Leg	Kaki
Liver	Hati/Liver

LOC or KO	Pingsan		Surgery	Operasi
Lungs	Paru-paru		Sweat	Keringat
			Swollen	Bengkak

M

Medicine	Obat		**T**	
Muscle	Otot		Tetanus	Tetanus
			This	Ini

N

Nausea	Mual		Throat	Tenggorokan
Nerve	Saraf		Thyroid	Tiroid
No	Tidak		Transfusion	Transfusi
Now	Sekarang		Tuberculosis	TBC
Nurse	Suster			

U

P			Ulcer	Ulcer
Pain	Sakit		Urine	Urin/Kencing
Please	Tolong			

V

Pneumonia	Pneumonia		Valve	Katup
Pressure	Tekanan		Vein	Vena
Pus	Nanah		Vomiting	Muntah

S

Same	Sama		**W**	
Sharp (pain)	Tajam		Want	Mau
Short breath	Susah nafas		Weak	Lemah
Shoulder	Bahu		Weakness	Kelemahan
Sick	Sakit		What	Apa
Small	Kecil		When	Kapan
Sorry	Maaf		Where	Dimana
Spine	Tulang punggung		Who	Siapa
Sputum	Gelama, Dahak		Worse	Memburuk
Start	Mulai			

X

Stomach	Perut		X-ray	X-ray
Stool	Tinja/Feses			

Y

Stop	Stop		Yes	Iya
Stroke	Stroke		You	Kamu
Strong	Kuat		Your	Anda

NUMBERS

one, two	ichi, ni
three, four	san, shi
five, six	go, roku

A

Abdomen	Hukubu/Onaka
Alcohol	Sake
Allergy	Alerugi
A little	Sukoshi
A lot	Takusan
Angiogram	Kekkanzouei
Anxiety	Shinpai
Appendix	Huroku
Appetite	Shokuyoku
Arm	Ude
Artery	Doumyaku
Arthritis	Kansetsuen

B

Back	Senaka/Ushiro
Bad	Warui
Better	Sarani-yoi
Big	Ooki
Blood	Ti/Ketueki
Brain	Nou
Breathe	Iki wo suru
Breathing	Kokyu
Burns	Yakedo

C

Cancer	Gan
Chest	Mune
Cough	Seki

D

Days	Nicchuwa
Defecation	Ben
Diabetes	Tounyoubyou
Disease	Byouki
Dizzy	Memaigashite
Doctor	Isha
Drink	Nomu/Nomimono

E

Ear	Mimi
Eat	Taberu
Elbow	Hiji
Eye	Me

F

Fever	Netu
Finger	Yubi
Foot	Ashi

G

Gallbladder	Tannou
Go	Ite
Good	Yoi

H

Hand	Te
Hard	Muzukashii
Have	Motsu
Head	Atama
Headache	Zutsuu
Heart	Sinzou
Heavy	Omoi
Help	Tasuke/Tasukeru
Here	Koko
Home	Ie
Hospital	Byouin
Hours	Jikan
How long	Donokurai
How many	Ikutsu
HTN	Kouketsuatsu

I

I, me	Wastashi wa
Injection	Chuusha
Intestines	Chou

K

Kidneys	Jinzou
Knee	Hiza

L

Lab tests	Jikken
Last	Saigo
Leg	Ashi

Liver	Kanzou		Strong	Tuyoi
LOC or KO	Ishiki-humei		Surgery	Geka/Shujutu
Lungs	Hai		Sweat	Amai
			Swollen	Hare

M

Medicine	Kusuri		**T**	
Muscle	Kin-niku		Tetanus	Hashouhuu
			This	Kore
N			Throat	Nodo
Nausea	Hakike		Thyroid	Koujousen
Nerve	Shinkei		Transfusion	Yuketu
No	Iie		Tuberculosis	Kekkaku
Now	Ima			
Nurse	Kangohu		**U**	
			Ulcer	Kaiyou
P			Urine	Nyou/Shouben
Pain	Itami			
Please	Douzo		**V**	
Pneumonia	Haien		Valve	Ben (maku)
Pressure	Atsuryoku/Kunou		Vein	Seimyaku
Pus	Umi, or noo		Vomit	Hakidasu
S			**W**	
Same	Onaji		Want	Husoku/Hituyou
Sharp (pain)	Surudoi		Weak	Yowai
Short breath	Ikigire		Weakness	Yowasa
Shoulder	Kata		What	Nani
Sick	Byouki		When	Itu
Small	Chiisai		Where	Doko
Sorry	Gomen nasai		Who	Dare
Spine	Sekichuu		Worse	Yoriwarui/Akka
Sputum	Tan			
Start	Hajimeru		**X**	
Stomach	I/Onaka		X-ray	Rentogen
Stool	Koshikake			
Stop	Yameru		**Y**	
Stroke	Nousocchuu		Yes	Hai
			You	Anata
			Your	Anatano

KOREAN (HANGUL)

NUMBERS

one, two	hana, dul
three, four	set, net
five, six	tassot, yossot

A

Abdomen	Bae
Alcohol	Sul
Allergy	Al-le-reu-gi
A little	Cho-geum
A lot	Mon-i
Angiogram	Yakmul shimchang chalyung
Anxiety	Keun shim
Appendicitis	Maeng-jang-yeom
Appetite	Shik-meok
Arm	P' al
Artery	Dong-mek
Arthritis	Kwonjulyum

B

Back	Deung
Bad	Na-ppeu- da
Better	Cho-a-yo
Big	Kun
Blood	P'i
Brain	Neo
Breathe	Seum shu
Breathing	Seum-shu-yo
Burns	Hwa-sang

C

Cancer	Aum
Chest	Ka-seum
Cough	Ki-ch'im

D

Days	Il/nal
Defecation	Taebyun
Diabetes	Dang neo byung
Disease	Beong
Dizzy	U-chi-lu-wu
Doctor	Eui-sa
Drink	Ma shyeo

E

Ear	Kwi
Eat	Meo-geo-yo
Elbow	P'al-kkum-ch'i
Eye	Nun (noon)

F

Fever	Yeoul
Finger	Son-kka-rak
Foot	Bal

G

Gallbladder	Sul gae
Go	Kada
Good	Ch-a-yo

H

Hand	Son
Hard	Ulu wa
Have	It-tta
Head	Meo ri
Headache	Meo-ri a peu
Heart	Shim-jang
heavy	Mu-geo-weo-yo
Help	To wa chu
Here	Yogi
Home	Chip
Hospital	Pyong Wan
Hours	Shigan
How long	Alma na
How many	Myopun
HTN	Kohyul op

I

I, me	Na
Injection	Chusa
Intestines	Jaong

K

Kidneys	Shin jang
Knee	Mu-reup

L

Lab tests	Hyulhek gumsa
Last	Ma-ji-mak
Leg	Ta-ri

Liver	Kan
LOC or KO	Usik bul myung
Lungs	Pae

M

Medicine	Yak
Muscle	Keun-yuk

N

Nausea	Me sik gu'um
Nerve	Shin keung
No	A-ni
Now	Chi-geum
Nurse	Kan-no-sa

P

Pain	A peu
Please	Che-bal
Pneumonia	Peyeum
Pressure	Amyuk
Pus	Iltahap

S

Same	Ka'tim
Sharp (pain)	A peu
Short breath	Sum ga pum
Shoulder	Eo-kkae
Sick	Pyeong-i
Small	Chak kum
Sorry	Myen hamnida
Spine	Ch'eok-ch'u
Sputum	Chim
Start	Sui-jak
Stomach	Wi jang
Stool	Dong
Stop	Se-weo-yo
Stroke	Ma bi/Sutu rok

Strong	Kang-ha-da Surgery su-sool
Sweat	Tam
Swollen	Pu'ota

T

Tetanus	Kwa sang
This	Yogi
Throat	Mok—kku-meong
Thyroid	Kap-sang sun
Transfusion	Suew heul
Tuberculosis	Pae gyul hek

U

Ulcer	Wi-gue-yang
Urine	O-jume

V

Valve	Mak
Vein	Cheung mek
Vomiting	Tow-he-yo

W

Want	Weon-ha-da
Weak	Yak-k'a-da
Weakness	Yak-he
What	Muot
When	Eon-je
Where	Eo-di
Who	Nu-gu
Worse	Dun a-ppeu

X

X-ray	X-ray

Y

Yes	Ne
You	Nu
Your	Neo-ku

PERSIAN (FARSI)

NUMBERS

one, two	yek, do
three, four	seem chahar
five, six	panj, shish

A

Abdomen	Shekam
Alcohol	Alcol
Allergy	Hasosiat
A little	Yek Zareh
A lot	Khaily
Angiogram	Angiogram
Anxiety	Ezterob
Appendix	Upondeese
Appetite	Mail Beh Ghaza
Arm	Bazu
Artery	Shah Rag
Arthritis	Arthrose

B

Back	Posht
Bed	Takht
Better	Behtar
Big	Bozorg
Blood	Khoon
Brain	Maghz
Breathe	Nafas Bekesh
Breathing	Nafas Keshidan
Burns	Sookhtegui

C

Cancer	Saraton
Chest	Seeneh
Cough	Sorfeh

D

Days	Rooz
Defecation	Tooalet kardan
Diabetes	Marazeh Ghand
Disease	Bimari
Dizzy	Sar Geejeh
Doctor	Doctor
Drink	Nooshidan

E

Ear	Goosh
Eat	Khordan
Elbow	Arenje
Eye	Cheshm

F

Fever	Tab
Finger	Angosht
Foot	Pa

G

Gallbladder	Kiseyeh Safra
Go	Berin
Good	Khoob

H

Hand	Dast
Hard/heavy	Sakht/Sangin
Have	Darid
Head	Sar
Headache	Sar Dard
Heart	Ghalb
Help	Komak
Here	INJA
Home	Khoone
Hospital	Bi Marestan
Hours	Sa At
How long	Chand Vaght
How many	Chand Ta
HTN	Feshare Khoon

I

I, me	Man
Injection	Ampool
Intestines	Roodeh

K

Kidneys	Kolieh
Knee	Zanu

L

Lab tests	Javobeh Azmayesh
Last	Aukhar
Leg	Pa

Liver	Jeegar
LOC or KO	Be hooshy
Lungs	Riye

M

Medicine	Dava
Muscle	Mahicheh

N

Nausea	Tahavoh
Nerve	Asab
No	Naa
Now	Al-on
Nurse	Parastar

P

Pain	Dard
Please	Khahesh Mikonam
Pneumonia	Sineh Pahloo
Pressure	Feshar
Pus	Au zard

S

Same	Hameentor
Sharp (pain)	Teer Mikesheh
Short breath	Nafas Tangeh
Shoulder	Shooneh
Sick	Mariz
Small	Koocheeck
Sorry	Be Bakhshin
Spine	Sotuneh Fagharat
Sputum	Khelt
Start	Av-val
Stomach	Medeh
Stool	Madfoo
Stop	Nakon
Stroke	Sektehe Maghzee

Strong	Ghavi
Surgery	Jarohe
Sweat	Aragh
Swollen	Pundi dagi

T

Tetanus	Kozuz
This	In
Throat	Galoo
Thyroid	Teroeed
Transfusion	Tazrige Khoon
Tuberculosis	Sel

U

Ulcer	Zakhmeh Medeh
Urine	Edrar

V

Valve	Daricheh
Vein	Rag
Vomiting	Estefrogh

W

Want	Khostan
Weak	Zaif
Weakness	Zaf
What	Chee
When	Kay
Where	Koja
Who	Key
Worse	Badtar

X

X-ray	Akse xray

Y

Yes	Baleh
You	Shoma
Your	Moleh Shoma

PHILIPPINO (TAGALOG)

NUMBERS

one, two	isa, dalawa
three, four	tatlo, apat
five, six	lima, anim

A

Abdomen	Tiyan/Sikmura
Alcohol	Alkohol
Allergy	Allergy
A little	Konti
A lot	Masyado
Angiogram	Angiogram
Anxiety	Nerbiyos
Appendix	Appendix
Appetite	Gana
Arm	Braso
Artery	Ugat
Arthritis	Rayuma

B

Back	Likod
Bad	Masama
Better	Mas mabuti
Big	Malaki
Blood	Dugo
Brain	Utak
Breathe	Hinga
Breathing	Hininga
Burns	Paso`

C

Cancer	Kancer
Chest	Dibdib
Cough	Ubo

D

Days	Araw
Defecation	Ta'e
Diabetes	Diabetes
Disease	Sakit
Dizzy	Hilo
Doctor	Doktor
Drink	Inom

E

Ear	Tenga
Eat	Kain
Elbow	Siko
Eye	Mata

F

Fever	Lagnat
Finger	Daliri
Foot	Paa

G

Gallbladder	Bato
Go	Punta
Good	Mabuti

H

Hand	Kamay
Hard/heavy	Matigas/mabigat
Have	Meron
Head	Ulo
Headache	Sakit ng ulo
Heart	Puso
Help	Tulong
Here	Dito
Home	Bahay
Hospital	Ospital
Hours	Oras
How long	Ga'ano katagal
How many	Ilan
HTN	Alta presyon

I

I, me	Ako
Injection	Ineksyon

K

Kidneys	Bato
Knee	Tuhod

L

Lab tests	Resultas
Last	Huli
Leg (low/high)	Binti/hita
Liver	Atay
LOC or KO	Nawalan ng malay
Lungs	Baga

M

Medicine	Gamot
Muscle	Masel

N

Nausea	Nasusuka
Nerve	Ugat
No	Hindi
Now	Ngayon
Nurse	Nurse

P

Pain	Masakit
Please	Paki
Pneumonia	Pulmonya
Pressure	Presyo
Pus	Pisga

S

Same	Pareho
Sharp (pain)	Makirot
Short breath	Nahirapang huminga
Shoulder	Balikat
Sick	Sakit
Small	Maliit
Sorry	Patawad
Spine	Gulugod
Sputum	Plema
Start	Umpisa
Stomach	Tiyan/Sikmura
Stool	Tae
Stop	Hinto
Stroke	Stroke
Strong	Malakas
Surgery	Operasyon
Sweat	Pawis
Swollen	Maga

T

Tetanus	Tetano
This	Ito
Throat	Ngala-ngala
Thyroid	Thyroid
Transfusion	Salinan ng dugo
Tuberculosis	TB

U

Ulcer	Ulser
Urine	Ihi

V

Valve	Balbula
Vein	Ugat
Vomiting	Suka

W

Want	Gusto
Weak	Mahina
Weakness	Kahinaan
What	Ano
When	Kailan
Where	Saan
Who	Sino
Worse	Mas malala

X

X-ray	X-ray

Y

Yes	Oo
You	Ikaw
Your	Sa iyo

POLISH (POLSKI) Note: R's are rolled

NUMBERS

one, two	yeden, dva
three, four	tshe, chtere
five, six	piench, sheshch

A

Abdomen	Bzhuh
Alcohol	Alkohol
Allergy	Alergia
A little	Trohe
A lot	Duzho
Anxiety	Nyepokooy
Appendix	Verostek
Appetite	Apetit
Arm	Renka
Artery	Tentneetza
Arthritis	Zapalenye stavoof

B

Back	Pletzy
Bad	Zhle
Better	Lepyey
Big	Duzhe
Blood	Kref
Brain	Moozk
Breathe	Oddehay
Breathing	Oddeh
Burns	Spalenye

C

Cancer	Rak
Chest	Klatka pyershova
Cough	Kashel

D

Days	Dnee
Defecation	Oddanye stoltza
Diabetes	Tzuksheetza
Disease	Horoba
Dizzy	Zavroty gwovy
Doctor	Doktor
Drink	Piy (to drink)

E

Ear	Uho
Eat	Yeshch
Elbow	Wokyech
Eye	Oko

F

Fever	Goronchka
Finger	Paletz
Foot	Stopa

G

Go	Ich
Good	Dobre

H

Hand	Dwon
Hard/heavy	Tvarde/chenshkye
Have	Mam, mash
Head	Gwova
Headache	Bool gwovy
Heart	Sertze
Help	Pomus
Here	Tutiy
Home	Dom
Hospital	Shpeetal
Hours	Godzheeni
How long	Yak dwoogo
How many	Eele

I

I, me	Ya, mee
Injection	Zastshik
Intestines	Yeleeta

K

Kidneys	Nerkee
Knee	Kolano

L

Lab tests	Badanya
Last	Ostatnye
Leg	Noga
Liver	Vontroba
LOC or KO	Stracheech pshetomnoshch
Lungs	Pwootza

M

Medicine	Lekarstvo
Muscle	Myenshen

N

Nausea	Noodnoshchee
Nerve	Nerva
No	Nye
Now	Teraz
Nurse	Pyelengyarka

P

Pain	Bool
Please	Proshe
Pneumonia	Zapalenye pwootz
Pressure	Cheeshnyenye
Pus	Ropa

S

Same	Takye sa-me
Sharp (pain)	Ostre
Short breath	Krootkee oddeh
Shoulder	Bark
Sick	Hory
Small	Mawe
Sorry	Psheprasham
Spine	Krengoswoop
Sputum	Shleena
Start	Start
Stomach	Zhowondek
Stool	Stoletz
Stop	Stop
Stroke	Velev krvee
Strong	Motzne
Surgery	Operatzya
Sweat	Pot
Swollen	Spuhniente

T

Tetanus	Tenzhetz
This	To
Throat	Gardwo
Thyroid	Tarchetza
Transfusion	Transfuzya
Tuberculosis	Groozhleetza

U

Ulcer	Vzhood
Urine	Moch

V

Valve	Zastavka
Vein	Zhewa
Vomiting	Vemyote

W

Want	Htze
Weak	Swabo
Weakness	Swaboshch
What	Tzo
When	Kyede
Where	Gdzye
Who	Kto
Worse	Gozhey

X

X-ray	Psheshvietlenie

Y

Yes	Tak
You	Ti
Your	Tvooy

PORTUGUESE

NUMBERS

one, two	um, dois,
three, four	tres quarto
five, six	cinco, seis

A

Abdomen	Estomago
Alcohol	Alcool
Allergy	Alergia
A little	Pouco
A lot	Muito
Anxiety	Nervos
Appendix	Apendice
Appetite	Apetito
Arm	Braco
Artery	Atreria
Arthritis	Artritis

B

Back	Costas
Bad	Ruim
Better	Melhor
Big	Grande
Blood	Sangue
Brain	Cerebro
Breathe	Respirar
Breathing	Respiracao
Burns	Arde, doi

C

Cancer	Cancer
Chest	Peito
Cough	Tos

D

Days	Dias
Defecation	Defecar
Diabetes	Diabetes
Disease	Enfermidad
Dizzy	Tonto, mariado
Doctor	Doctor
Drink	Bebida

E

Ear	Orelha
Eat	Coma! comer
Elbow	Cortevelo
Eye	Olho

F

Fever	Fevre
Finger	Dedo
Foot	Pie

G

Gallbladder	Vesicula
Go	Ir, va!
Good	Bom

H

Hand	Mao
Hard/heavy	Pesado
Have	Ter
Head	Cabeza
Headache	Dolor de cabeza
Heart	Corazon
Help	Ayuda
Here	Aqui
Home	Casa
Hospital	Hospital
Hours	Horas
How long	Quanto Tempo
How many	Quantos?
HTN	Ipertensao

I

I, Me	Eu, Mim
Injection	Injeção
Intestines	Intestinos

K

Kidneys	Rims
Knee	Joelho

L

Lab tests	Analysis de sangre
Last	Ultima
Leg	Pierna
Liver	Figado
LOC or KO	Perdidoconciencia
Lungs	Pulmones

M

Medicine	Medicina
Muscle	Musculo

N

Nausea	Nausea, agrudas
Nerve	Nervio
No	Nao
Now	Agora
Nurse	Enfermera

P

Pain	Dor
Please	Por favor
Pneumonia	Pneumonia
Pressure	Pressio

S

Same	Mesmo
Sharp (pain)	Agudo
Short Breath	Falta de aire
Shoulder	Hombro
Sick	Doente
Small	Pequeno
Sorry	Desculpe
Spine	Espina
Sputum	Flemas
Start	Comecar
Stomach	Estomago
Stool	Defecacion
Stop	Parar
Stroke	Embolio
Strong	Forte
Surgery	Cirugia

Sweat	Suar
Swollen	Inflamado

T

Tetanus	Tetano
This	Este
Throat	Garganta
Thyroid	Tiroides
Transfusion	Transfusion
Tuberculosis	Tuberculosis

U

Ulcer	Ulcera
Urine	Orina

V

Valve	Valvula
Vein	Vena
Vomiting	Vomitos

W

Want	Querer
Weak	Fraco
Weakness	Fraquesa
What	Que?
When	Cuando
Where	Donde
Who	Quem
Worse	Pior

X

X-ray	Haiyo shish

Y

Yes	Sim
You	Voce
Your	Seu-sua

RUSSIAN (RUSKI)

NUMBERS

one, two	odin, dva
three, four	tri, chetire
five, six	pyat, shest

A

Abdomen	Ghivot
Alcohol	Alcogol
Allergy	Allerghia
A little	Chuchut
A lot	Mnoga
Angiogram	Angiograma
Anxiety	Trevoga
Appendix	Apendix
Appetite	Apetit
Arm	Ruka
Artery	Arteria
Arthritis	Artrit

B

Back	Spina
Bad	Ploho
Better	Ludshe
Big	Bolshoy
Blood	Krov
Brain	Mozg
Breathe	Deshi
Breathing	Dehanye
Burns	Pechot

C

Cancer	Rak
Chest	Grud
Cough	Kashel

D

Days	D'ni
Defecation	Kal, Stool
Diabetes	Diabet
Disease	Baleznye
Dizzy	Kruzhitsa golova
Doctor	Doctor
Drink	Peet

E

Ear	Uho
Eat	Kushat
Elbow	Lokot
Eye	Glaz

F

Fever	Temperatura
Finger	Paletz
Foot	Stupnya

G

Gallbladder	Zhelchnye Puzur
Go	Davaj, Idti
Good	Harasho

H

Hand	Ruka
Hard/heavy	Tyaghelo
Have	Imet
Head	Golova
Headache	Bolit Golova
Heart	Certze
Help	Pamagatz
Here	Zdes
Home	Dom
Hospital	Bolnitsa
Hours	Chasi
How long	Kak dolgo
How many	Skolko
HTN	Visokoe davlenie

I

I, me	Ya
Injection	Ukol
Intestines	Kishki

K

Kidneys	Pochkie
Knee	Koleno

L

Lab tests	Analiz
Last	Poslednie
Leg	Noga
Liver	Pecheyn

LOC or KO	Poteryat soznanie		Surgery	Operatzi
Lungs	Leghie		Sweat	Pot
			Swollen	Opukhshee
M				
Medicine	Lekarstvo		**T**	
Muscle	Muskul		Tetanus	Privivka
			This	Eto
N			Throat	Gorlo
Nausea	Tashnit		Thyroid	Schitovitka
Nerve	Nyerve		Transfusion	Perelivaniye
No	Nyet		Tuberculosis	Tuberculos
Now	Sechast			
Nurse	Med sestra		**U**	
			Ulcer	Yazva
P			Urine	Mocha
Pain	Balit			
Please	Poshalsta		**V**	
Pneumonia	Pneuvmonia		Valve	Valva
Pressure	Davlenie		Vein	Vena
Pus	Gnoj		Vomiting	Rvota
S			**W**	
Same	Odinakoviy		Want	Hotet
Sharp (pain)	Kolit		Weak	Slabie
Short breath	Otdishka		Weakness	Slabost
Shoulder	Plecho		What	Chto
Sick	Bolet		When	Kogda
Small	Malenky		Where	G'de
Sorry	Izvinite		Who	Kto
Spine	Pazvanochnik		Worse	Huzhe
Sputum	Makrota			
Start	Nachat		**X**	
Stomach	Zhivot		X-ray	Rengen
Stool	Kal			
Stop	Stop		**Y**	
Stroke	Insult		Yes	Da
Strong	Silno		You	Vee
			Your	Vashe

SPANISH (ESPAÑOL, CASTELLANO)

NUMBERS

one, two	uno, dos
three, four	tres, quatro
five, six	cinquo, seis

A

Abdomen	Abdomen
Alcohol	Alcohol
Allergy	Allergia
A little	Poco/Poquito
A lot	Mucho
Angiogram	Angiograma
Anxiety	Nervios
Appendix	Appendice
Appetite	Apetito
Arm	Brazo
Artery	Arteria
Arthritis	Artritis

B

Back	Espalda
Bed	Cama
Better	Mejor
Big	Grande
Blood	Sangre
Brain	Cerebro
Breathe	Respira
Breathing	Respiracion
Burn	Arde, Quemada

C

Cancer	Cancer
Chest	Pecho
Cough	Tos

D

Days	Dias
Defecation	Popo
Diabetes	Diabetes
Disease	Enfermedad
Dizzy	Mareos
Doctor	Doctor
Drink	Toma

E

Ear	Oido
Eat	Come
Elbow	Codo
Eye	Ojo

F

Fever	Fiebre
Finger	Dedo
Foot	Pie

G

Gallbladder	Vesicula
Go	Valla
Good	Bueno

H

Hand	Mano
Hard/heavy	Duro/Pesado
Have	Tiene
Head	Cabeza
Headache	Dolor de Cabeza
Heart	Corazon
Help	Ayuda
Here	Aqui
Home	Casa
Hospital	Hospital
Hours	Horas
How long	Cuantos horas
How many	Cuantos
HTN	Presion Alta

I

I, me	Yo, me
Injection	Injecion
Intestines	Intestinos

J

Joint	Collontura

K

Kidneys	Rinones
Knee	Rodilla

L

Lab tests	Analysis de sangre
Last	Ultima
Leg	Pierna
Liver	Higado
LOC or KO	Perdida de conciencia
Lungs	Pulmones

M

Medicine	Medicina
Muscle	Musculo

N

Nausea	Nausea, agruras
Nerve	Nervio
No	No
Now	Ahorita
Nurse	Enfermera

P

Pain	Dolor
Please	Por Favor
Pneumonia	Pneumonia
Pressure	Presion
Pus	Pus

S

Same	Mismo
Sharp (pain)	Agudo
Short breath	Falta de aire
Shoulder	Hombro
Sick	Enfermo
Small	Pequeno
Sorry	Lo siento
Spine	Espina
Sputum	Flemas/esputo
Start	Empeiza
Stomach	Estomago
Stool	Defecacion
Stop	Para

Stroke	Embolio
Strong	Fuerte
Surgery	Cirugia
Sweat	Sudar
Swollen	Hinchado

T

Tetanus	Tetano
This	Este
Throat	Garganta
Thyroid	Tiroides
Transfusion	Transfusion
Tuberculosis	Tuberculosis

U

Ulcer	Ulcera
Urine	Orina

V

Valve	Valvula
Vein	Vena
Vomiting	Vomitos

W

Want	Queire
Weak	Debil
Weakness	Debilidad
What	Que
When	Cuando
Where	Donde
Who	Quien
Worse	Peor

X

X-ray	Radiografia

Y

Yes	Si
You	Usted
Your	Su

TURKISH

NUMBERS

one, two	bir, iki
three, four	ug, dort
five, six	besh, alti

A

Abdomen	Karin
Alcohol	Alkol/Ichki
Allergy	Alerji
A little	Az/Ufak
A lot	Chok
Angiogram	Angiogram
Anxiety	Heves
Appendix	Apandis
Appetite	Ishtah
Arm	Kol
Artery	Atardamar
Arthritis	Romatizmo

B

Back	Arka
Bad	Fena/Kotu
Better	Daha iyi/guzel
Big	Buyuk
Blood	Kan
Brain	Beyin
Breathe	Nefes Alip
Breathing	Bir nefes lik
Burns	Yanik

C

Cancer	Kanser
Chest	Guose
Cough	Uksurmek

D

Days	Gune
Defecation	Sigmak
Diabetes	Diabet
Disease	Enfermidad
Dizzy	Bash
Doctor	Doktor
Drink	Ichmek

E

Ear	Kulak
Eat	Yemek
Elbow	Dirsek
Eye	Goz/Guz

F

Fever	Atesh
Finger	Parmak
Foot	Ayak

G

Gallbladder	Safra kesesi
Go	Git
Good	Iyi, Guzel

H

Hand	El
Hard/heavy	Zor/Ahir
Have	Sahip Ol/Olmak
Head	Bash
Headache	Bash Ahrisi
Heart	Kalp
Help	Yardim
Here	Burada
Home	Ev
Hospital	Hastane
Hours	Saatler
How long	Ne kadar
How many	Kag tane
HTN	Yuksek tensiyon

I

I, me	Ben
Injection	Injeksiyon
Intestines	Bahirsaklar

K

Kidneys	Bubrek
Knee	Diz

L

Lab tests	Laboratuvar
Last	Son
Leg	Bajak

Liver	Karajiher
LOC or KO	Senkop/Bayhinlik
Lungs	Akjiher

M

Medicine	Ilach
Muscle	Pazi

N

Nausea	Mide Bulantisi
Nerve	Sinir
No	Hayer Hich
Now	Shimdi/Hemen
Nurse	Hemshire

P

Pain	Ahri
Please	Rejha Ederem
Pneumonia	Zaturree
Pressure	Basich
Pus	Iltahap

S

Same	Ayni
Sharp (pain)	Sivri
Short breath	Alchak Nefes
Shoulder	Omuz
Sick	Hasta
Small	Ufak/Kuchuk
Sorry	Ozur
Spine	Kilchik
Sputum	Salya/Balgam
Start	Bashlama
Stomach	Karin
Stool	Kaka
Stop	Durma
Stroke	Felch
Strong	Guchlu

Surgery	Ameliyatane
Sweat	Ter
Swollen	Shishik

T

Tetanus	Tetanos
This	Bu
Throat	Bohaz/Girtlak
Thyroid	Tiroid
Transfusion	Kan Nakli
Tuberculosis	Verem

U

Ulcer	Ulser
Urine	Chish

V

Valve	Valf
Vein	Damar
Vomiting	Kusma

W

Want	Istemek
Walking	Yurumek
Weak	Kuvvetsis
Weakness	Kuvvetsizlik
What	Ne
When	Nezaman
Where	Nerede
Who	Kim/Kimi
Worse	Daha Kotu

X

X-ray	Rontgen

Y

Yes	Evet
You	Sen
Your	Senin

VIETNAMESE (TIENG VIETNAM)

NUMBERS

one, two	mot, hai
three, four	ba, bon
five, six	nam, sau

A

Abdomen	Bung
Alcohol	Ruou
Allergy	Di Ung
A little	Mot chut
A lot	Nhieu
Angiogram	Chieu cach tim
Anxiety	Lo lang/Hoi hop
Appendix	Ruot du
Appetite	Khau vi
Arm	Canh tay
Artery	Mach mau
Arthritis	Dau khop xuong

B

Back	Lung
Bad	Xau/Khong tot
Better	Kha hon
Big	Lon
Blood	Mau
Brain	Oc
Breathe	Tho
Breathing	Hoi tho
Burns	Phong

C

Cancer	Ung thu
Chest	Long nguc
Cough	Ho

D

Days	Ngay
Defecation	Di cau
Diabetes	Tieu duong
Disease	Benh
Dizzy	Chong mat
Doctor	Bac si
Drink	Uong

E

Ear	Tai
Eat	An
Elbow	Khuyu cho
Eye	Mat

F

Fever	Sot, nong
Finger	Ngon tay
Foot	Chan

G

Gallbladder	La Lach
Go	Di
Good	Tot

H

Hand	Tay
Hard/heavy	Nang nhoc
Have	Co
Head	Dau
Headache	Nhuc dau
Heart	Tim
Help	Giup
Here	O day
Home	Nha
Hospital	Behn vien
Hours	Gio
How long	Bao lau
How many	Bau nhieu
HTN	Cau mau

I

I, me	Toi
Injection	Chit
Intestines	Ruot

K

Kidneys	Than
Knee	Dau goi

L

Lab tests	Thu mau
Last	Cuoi cung
Leg	Chan, cang

Liver	Gan	Surgery	Giai phau
LOC or KO	Xiu	Sweat	Mo hoi
Lungs	Phoi	Swollen	Sung

M

T

Medicine	Thuoc	Tetanus	Uon van
Muscle	Bap thit	This	Cai nay

N

		Throat	Co hong
Nausea	Buon non, mua	Thyroid	Yet hau
Nerve	Giay than kinh	Transfusion	Truyen mau
No	Khong	Tuberculosis	Benh Lao
Now	Bay gio		
Nurse	Y ta		

U

P

		Ulcer	Ung nhot/Luyet
Pain	Dau	Urine	Nuoc tieu
Please	Lam on		

V

Pneumonia	Xung phoi	Valve	Ong dan
Pressure	Suc de nang	Vein	Mach mau
Pus	Mu	Vomiting	Non mua

S

W

Same	Giong nhau	Want	Muon
Sharp (pain)	Dau dieng	Weak	Yeu
Short breath	Tho doc	Weakness	Su suy yeu
Shoulder	Vai	What	Cai gi
Sick	Dau om	When	Khi, luc nao
Small	Nho	Where	O dau
Sorry	Xin loi	Who	Ai
Spine	Xuong song	Worse	Xau hon

Sputum	Dom

X

Start	Bat dau	X-ray	Jub Hun
Stomach	Bao tu		

Y

Stool	Phan	Yes	Co, Da
Stop	Ngung	You	Ong, ba, co, em
Stroke	Tai bien mach mau	Your	Cua ong, ba, co
Strong	Manh		

QUICK REFERENCE

DECODING AND DDX OF ABNORMAL VITAL SIGNS

- **BP**
  - *High*: Spurious, essential HTN, secondary HTN (endocrine, renal artery stenosis, drugs)
  - *Low*: Pay attention to diastolic BP. JVD? Clear lungs? Murmur? Kussmaul? (See "Shock" section here)
  - *Wide*: Pulse pressure: "PAST" (PDA, AI, AV fistula, Sepsis, TSH); Also coarctation
- **Bilateral BP**: Important to check in hypotension as well: the higher of the two arms is the true BP; 20% of normal people will have a 20 mmHg difference in the SBP.
- **Orthostatics**: Don't do if patient already symptomatic: risk outweighs benefit; low sensitivity and specificity; "positive" if SBP < 90 or drop > 25 or HR ↑ by >30.
  - *DDx*: Hypovolemia, autonomic dysfunction, meds, normal variant
- **Pulse**
  - *Fast*: ↑: **T**ox (e.g.: coke, antichol), **T**wist (pain or anxiety), **T**SH/pheo, **T**emp. (↑1°F > HR↑ by 10).
    ↓: Blood (anemia, BP, volume, heart), O_2 (PE, CHF), EtOH (withdrawal), glucose↓
  - *Slow*: ↑: ↑K, ↑Mg, ↑↑TSH, ↑Trop, ↑tox (BB, CCB, clonidine, digoxin, physostigmine, cyanide).
    ↓: ↓temperature, ↓O_2, ↓glucose, ↓conduction (AVB, SSS)
- **Temp.**
  - *Hot*: ID, TSH, CVD, CA (blood, L, K, lung, prostate), tox (NMS, cocaine, antichol), heat stroke
  - *Cold*: Exposure, sepsis, TSH (neck scar), hypoglycemia; 37.8 = 100
- **Resps**
  - *High*: Sepsis, hypoxia, PE, CHF, RAD, ASA, TSH, anxiety, acidosis
  - *Low*: Drug (opiate, benzo, etc.), CNS

SHOCK: MAP MOST IMPORTANT: KEEP 65–75. IF NO IMPROVEMENT AFTER 2L NS, GIVE BLOOD OR PRESSORS.

- **Bilateral BP**: The higher of the two arms is the true BP.
- **JVD + Clear Lung**: PE, TPTX, tamponade, RVMI, RVCHF, constrictive CM or pericarditis
- **ED Echo**: IVC: Volume. RV dilatation: PE. Wall motion: AMI. RV collapse: tamponade.
- **Hypovolemic**: DDx: Bleed, dehydration; Rx: IVF, blood, surgery
- **Obstructive**: DDx: PE, PTX, tamp.; Rx: Heparin or needle
- **Cardiogenic**: DDx: CHF, MI, CM, meds; Rx: SBP: > 80: dobutamine; < 80: DA; < 70: NE, IABP
- **Distributive**: DDx: Sepsis, Addison's; Rx: IVF > (replete calcium) > (steroid) > pressors

TABLE A.1. Pediatric Vital Signs

Formula (Age in Years)	0 yr	1 yr	2 yr	4 yr	8 yr
Weight in Kilos = 10 + 2 (age) or 4 + (months/2)	4–10 kg	10 kg	14 kg	18 kg	26 kg
Max normal HR = 170 − 10 (age)	170	160	150	130	90
Min normal BP = 70 + 2 (age)	70	72	74	78	86
Max normal RR = 50 − 10 (age)	50	40	30	25	20

(Formula break down as age↑. Every book has different values.)
Source: Pregerson, DB. *Quick Essentials Emergency Medicine 4.0.* ERpocketbooks.com; 2010:160.

DICTATION TEMPLATES

ED BASIC H&P DICTATION

■ **General:** Patient name and ID. Date and time of arrival. Mode of arrival. MD time
■ **H&P:** HPI, PMH, PSH, meds, allergies, SH, ROS; vital signs, exam
■ **Tests:** EKG, plain films, blood work, UA and other lab, CT, US, special tests
■ **Course:** Treatment and response, consults, other interventions
■ **MDM:** Medical decision making: differential diagnosis, reasoning, treatments
■ **Dispo:** Impression, condition, disposition; aftercare, restrictions, Rx, follow-up

WORKERS COMP DICTATION*

Doctor's first report, California. Include employer, location, time, and date of injury. Does company require drug screen?

17. Patient description of events
18. Subjective complaints
19. Objective: Exam and tests
20. Diagnosis: Toxins: Y/N
21. Findings consistent: Y/N**

22. Delay in recovery: Y**/N
23. Treatment rendered
24. Further Rx required: Y**/N
25. Admission? If so, location?
26. Work: Off/Modified/Regular

* Patients with workers' comp and nonworkers' comp issues need two charts.

**Please explain and give dates where applicable.

WORKERS COMP PROGRESS REPORT, CALIFORNIA

■ **Types of Reports:** Periodic, change in work status, change in Rx plan, discharged, other; Include: employer, treatment plan and work status

CENTRAL LINE PROCEDURE NOTE: "SCUBA"

■ **Basics**: Indication: (no IV access, shock, hemodialysis). Consent: (from patient, family, implied)
S: Site (The _____ SITE was selected due to lung disease, DVT, patient request, orthopnea, etc.)
C: Cleaning (Skin was cleansed and prepared with CHLORHEXIDINE)
U: US (ULTRASOUND was used to locate the vein, cannulate vein)
B: Barriers (Wide field sterile BARRIERS were established and maintained throughout the procedure)
A: Antibiotic (An ANTIBIOTIC-coated _____ catheter was inserted over a guide wire)
■ **Complication**: Complications were _____. All ports drew blood and were flushed with saline.

ED INTRAVENOUS HYDRATION NOTE

■ **Infusion**: "Under my supervision, the patient received _____ ml of _____ IV fluid over _____ hours."
■ **Indication**: "IV fluids were indicated due to _____" (vomiting, dehydration, low BP, shock, sepsis)
■ **Re-assess**: "Clinical status and vital sign improvement noted following IV infusion."

RESOURCES

SELECTED RESOURCES

DRUGS

Lacy CF, Armstrong LL, Goldman MP, Lance LL, eds. *Drug Information Handbook 2010–2011: A Comprehensive Resource for All Clinicians and Healthcare Professionals*. 19th ed. Hudson, OH: Lexi-Comp; 2010.

Pregerson DB. *A to Z Pocket Pharmacopoeia*. 2nd ed. ERpocketbooks.com; 1996.

EKGs

Dubin D. *Rapid Interpretation of EKG's*. 6th ed. Tampa, FL: COVER, Inc.; 2000.

Surawicz B, Knilans TK. *Chou's Electrocardiography in Clinical Practice: Adult and Pediatric*. 6th ed. Philadelphia: Saunders; 2008.

EMERGENCY MEDICINE

Pregerson DB. *Quick Essentials: Emergency Medicine* 4.0. ERpocketbooks.com; 2010.

Tintanelli JE, Kelen GD, Stapczynski JS. *Emergency Medicine: A Comprehensive Study Guide*. 6th ed. New York: McGraw-Hill; 2003.

HISTORY AND PHYSICAL EXAM

Bickley LS, Szilagyi PG. *Bates' Guide to Physical Examination and History Taking*. 10th ed. Philadelphia: Lippincott Williams & Wilkins; 2008.

Ferri FF. *Practical Guide to the Care of the Medical Patient*. 8th ed. Philadelphia: Mosby, Inc.; 2011.

Goldberg S, Ouellette H. *Clinical Anatomy Made Ridiculously Simple*. 4th ed. Miami, FL: MedMaster, Inc.; 2010.

LAB

Gomella LG, Haist SA. *Clinician's Pocket Reference (Scut Monkey)*. 11th ed. New York: McGraw-Hill Medical; 2006.

MED-LEGAL

Leebov W, Vergare M, Scott G. *Patient Satisfaction: A Guide to Practice Enhancement*. Los Angeles: Practice Management Information Corporation; 1990.

MEDICINE

Fauci AS, Braunwald E, Kasper DL, et al. *Harrison's Principles of Internal Medicine*. 17th ed. New York: McGraw-Hill Medical; 2008.

Wolff K, Johnson RA. *Fitzpatrick's Color Atlas and Synopsis of Clinical Dermatology*. 6th ed. New York: McGraw-Hill; 2009.

OB-GYN

DeCherney AH, Nathan L, Goodwin TM, Laufer N. *CURRENT Diagnosis & Treatment: Obstetrics & Gynecology*. 10th ed. New York: McGraw-Hill Medical; 2006.

Hacker NF, Gambone JC, Hobel CJ. *Hacker & Moore's Essentials of Obstetrics and Gynecology*. 5th ed. Philadelphia: Saunders; 2010.

ORTHOPEDICS

Birrer RB, O'Connor FG. *Sports Medicine for the Primary Care Physician*. 3rd ed. Boca Raton, FL: CRC Press; 2004.

Dandy DJ, Edwards DJ. *Essential Orthopaedics and Trauma*. 5th ed. New York: Churchill Livingstone; 2003.

PEDIATRICS

Crain E, Gershel J. *Clinical Manual of Emergency Pediatrics*. 5th ed. New York: Cambridge University Press; 2010.

Kliegman R, Behrman RE, Nelson WE, Jenson HB. *Nelson Textbook of Pediatrics*. 18th ed. Philadelphia: Saunders; 2007.

PROCEDURES

Dunmire SM, Paris PM. *Atlas of Emergency Procedures*. Philadelphia: Saunders; 1994.

Roberts JR, Hedges JR. *Clinical Procedures in Emergency Medicine*. 5th ed. Philadelphia: Saunders; 2009.

RADIOLOGY

Basak S, Nazarian LN, Weschler RJ, et al. Is unenhanced CT sufficient for evaluation of acute abdominal pain? *Clin Imaging*. 2002; 26(6):405–407.

Picano E. Informed consent and communication of risk from radiological and nuclear medicine examinations: how to escape from a communication inferno. *BMJ*. 2004;329(7470):849–851.

Raby N, de Lacey G, Berman L. *Accident and Emergency Radiology: A Survival Guide*. Philadelphia: Saunders; 2005.

Simon BC, Snoey ER. *Ultrasound in Emergency and Ambulatory Medicine*. St. Louis, MO: Mosby; 1997.

Squire LF, Novelline RA. *Squire's Fundamentals of Radiology*. 6th ed. Cambridge, MA: Harvard University Press; 2004.

RESUSCITATION

Hazinski MF, Field JM, Gilmore D. *Handbook of Emergency Cardiovascular Care 2008: For Healthcare Providers*. Dallas, TX: American Heart Association; 2008.

SELECTED JOURNALS

Annals of Emergency Medicine	*Consultant Journal*	*Emergency Physicians Monthly*
The Clinical Advisor	*Emergency Medicine Magazine*	*New England Journal of Medicine*

PERSONAL "IN A PINCH" SPECIALIST PHONE LIST

SPECIALTY	UNDERINSURED	HMO	PPO
Allergy/immunology			
Cardiology			
Dermatology			
Endocrinology			
ENT			
General surgery			
Hematology			
ID			
Internal medicine			
Nephrology			
Neurology			
Neurosurgery			
Ophthalmology			
Orthopedic hand			
Orthopedics			
Plastic surgery			
Podiatry			
Pulmonary			
Rheumatology			
Urology			
Vascular surgery			

OTHER PHONE NUMBERS AND CONTACTS:

INDEX

Note: Page numbers followed by "f" and "t" denote figures and tables, respectively.

1° AV block 24
2° AV block 24
3 Ts 32
3° AV block 24, 132
4-lines 48
4 Ps 18
8-hr rule 93
72-hour hold 107

Aa gradient 30, 32
AAA 55, 56f
ABCs 50, 131
Abdomen 81
Abdominal CT 64
ABEM 127
ABGs 30, 32
Abnormal D/C vitals 102
Abnormal heart sounds 11t
Abruption 59
Absolute benefit 122
Abuse 110, 111
ABX 1st 98
Accelerated idio-ventricular rhythm 27
Accepting higher level of care transfers 108
Accepting lateral transfers 108
Accounting 128
ACE inhibitor 92, 136
Acetaminophen 40
Acid-base 32
Acid-base disorder 33
Acidosis 32
Acidotic conditions 32t
ACLS 2005 131
Acute coronary syndrome 22
Adenosine 23, 136
Adjustments 30
Admission decisions and bed type 106
Admission holding orders 106
Admissions 106
Adult epiglottitis 63f
Adult resuscitation 131–134
Aftercare 93
Age 18
Airspace 49
Airway 70–73, 137
Airway backups 70
Airway indications 70
Airway preparations 70
Albumin 17, 34
Alk phos 34
Alkalosis 32
Alkalotic conditions 32t
Allergies 2
ALT 34
AMA 104
Amio vs. lido 132
Amiodarone 29, 136
Ammonia 34
Amylase 34
Analgesia and driving 105
Analgesic comparison table 105t
Analgesics 105

Anaphylactoid 61
Anchoring 101
Anemia 36
Anesthesia 86
   extremities 94
   face 94
Anesthetic injections 93
Aneurysm 62, 64
Anion gap 30, 40
Anion gap acidosis labs 32
Ankle 52, 89, 91
Ankle relocation 91f
Anterior epistaxis 87
Antibiotics 93
Aorta 56f
Aorta technique 56
APGAR scores 139t
Appendicitis 58f, 64, 102
Apt test 42
Arbitration 117
Arm peripheral nerves 12
Arrythmias 137
Arterial thrombosis 60f
Arthritis 51
Arthrocentesis 89
   and joint injections 89
   results 89
   results by condition 89t
   sites 89
Artifacts 18
ASA class 99t
Assault 111
Assessment of practice performance 127
Asset protection 128
AST 34
Asystole 132
Asystole/PEA 137
Atrial ectopic tachycardia 26
Atrial fibrillation 26
Atrial flutter 26
Atropine 73, 136, 137
Attorney choosing 117
Atypical lymphocytes 37
Atypical Sx 102
AV block 24
Availability bias 101
Average glucose 33
Awake intubation 72

Backwards upwards rightwards pressure 72
Bacteria 41
Bacterial infection 25
Bag valve mask 70, 73, 74
Bandemia 37
Bariatrics 81
Barriers to return 102
Basal ganglia 62
Basophils 38
Behavioral issues 110
Beir block 92
Bell curve 30
Benadryl 93

Beta HCG 34, 41
Biases 121
Bicarb 136
Bi-level positive airway pressure 74
Biliary Dz 64
Bilirubin 34
Billing 101, 119–120
Billing levels for emergency department charting 119t
Bimanual intubation 71f, 72, 83
Bites 93
Bladder 64
Blades 137
Bleeding 62
Blood cultures 42
Blood draw 111
Blood pressure 4, 134
Bones 49
Bougie 73
Bounceback risks 102
Bradycardia 4, 24, 132, 137
Brain 85f
Brain natiuritic peptide 35
Breathing 74–76
Breech 83
Bronchospasm 11
Broselow Tape 138
Brugada syndrome 25
Buckle Fx 51
Bugs 93
Bulbocavernosus 14
BUN 31
Bupivicaine 93
Burnout 126
Buying 128

C-reactive protein 36
C-reactive protein and erythrocyte sedimentation rate 36
Calcaneus 52
Calcification 50, 51, 62
Calcium 31, 136
   high, low 28
California state and federal law 110–111
Call panel 108
Callous 51
Calorics 14
Canada tool 48
Cancer 47, 102
Canthotomy 86
Capacity 104
Cardiac anatomy 11f
Cardiac labs 35
Cardiac records 30
Cardiac sestamibi scans 65
Cardiac/mediastinum 49
Career, wellness, and finance 125–128
Casts 41
CBC 30
Cell count 89
Central lines 78, 79
Central nervous system 84–85

Cerebellar 14
Cerebrospinal fluid 85
Cervical spine CT 63
Cervical spine X-rays 48
Cesarian section 83
Charges (not costs) 17
Charting 111, 114–115
Chemistry 17, 30
Chest 75
Chest CT 63
Chest exam 11
Chest tube 75
Chest X-ray 75
Child Protective Services 107, 110
Chlamydia 44
Choking 131, 137
Cholesterol 35
Circulation 77–80
CK, total 35
CK labs 35
Cleaning 95
CMS 108, 111
CNS 134
Coagulation 39f
Coagulation tests 38
Cold agglutinin 43
Collapse 131
Combitube 70
Common bile duct 57
Communication 101
Comparative radiation doses
    from diagnostic imaging 46
Comparison bias 121
Comparison of test characteristics
    for coronary artery 66t
Compartment pressure
    measurement 88
Compartment syndrome and
    tendonitis 88
Competence 104
Complications 116
Composite endpoint 122
Computers 110
Confirmation bias 101
Confounders 121
Consent 36, 69
Consultants interaction 114
Consulting 117
Contaminant 41
Continuous certification exam 127
Contraband 111
Contrast 17
Contrast issue 61
Convict 111
Coordinating care 114
Core measures 106
Corneals 14
Coronary 63
Coronary CT angiography 66
Cortisol 34
Costs 17
Countershock levels for various
    dysrhythmias 131t
Court order 110, 111
Courtesy 126
CPR 131, 137
Cranial nerves 14
Crash ED Cesarian section 83
Creatinine 31
Cremasteric 14
Crichothyrotomy 73

Critical care 120
Crystals 41, 89
CSF D-dimer 85
CT scans 48, 51, 61–64
Culture results 43t
Cultures 42
CVP 78
Cystograms 82

D-dimer 35
DDx 4, 24, 85, 131
Dealing with complications 116
Dealing with errors 116
Death 109, 134, 137
Death telling 109, 134
Decels 83
Decision-making capacity 104
Declaring brain death 109
Deductions 128
Delayed 1° 95
Delivery 83
Delta-delta 33
Denial of care 120
Department of health services 107
Deposition 117, 118
Derm body map 9f
Dermabond 95
Devil's triangle 97
Diagnoses and pitfalls 101–102
Diagnostic errors and some causes 101
Diagnostic inertia 101
Diagnostic peritoneal lavage 81
Diagnostic terminology 120
Diaphragm 49
Difficult airway and failed airway 73
Diffuse axonal injury 62
Digibind 136
Digoxin 29, 40
Dilantin 40
Dilated aortic arch with dissection 56f
Dilated RV and RA from
    pulmonary embolism 55f
Dilation 77
Diltiazem 136
Direct fluorescent antibody 43
DISIDA 65
Disk space 48
Dislocations 90–91
    above the waist 90
    below the waist 91
Disposition—home 103, 104
Diverticulitis 64
DNA panel 42
DNR 109
Dobutamine 23, 136
Doctors 123
Dohle bodies 37f
Domestic violence 111
Dopamine 136
Double wall sign 50f
Downcodes 120
Dressing 97
Driving 105
Drug levels 40
Drugs and toxins 40
Drugs for wide complex
    tachydsrhythmias 133t
Duplex 66
Duty to third parties 116
DVT 60
Dystocia 83

Ear 97
Ear culture 42
Ear foreign body 87
Early termination 122
Ears 87
Echo technique 55
Echocardiogram 66
Ectopic 59
ED systems 114
ED systems and charting 114–115
ED top misses and common reasons 102
Edema 62
Effusion 11, 55
EKG 17, 18–29, 40, 120
Elbow 51, 89, 90
Elbow relocation 90
Elder or child abuse 111
Electricity 137
Electrolytes 28, 31
Electron beam CT 66
ELISA 43
Elopement 104
Email 114
Emancipated minors 110
Emergency medicine continuous
    certification 127
EMLA 93
EMTALA 108
End-of-shift bias 101
Endocrine 34
Enzyme-linked immunosorbent-assay 43
Eosinophils 37
Epidemics 1
Epinephrine 93, 136
Episiotomy 83
Epistaxis 87
Eponymous exam signs 7t
Errors 116
Erythrocyte sedimentation rate 36
Esmolol 136
ET tubes 137
Ethics: principles of proper conduct for
    given circumstances 116
EtOH 30
Event form 114
Excessive awards 118
Exercise stress tests and advanced
    cardiac evaluation 23
Expectation management 113
Experimental studies 121
Expert witnesses 118
Extended focus assessment with
    sonography in trauma 54
External validity 122
Eye anatomy 10f
Eye culture 42
Eye exam 10
Eyelid 97
Eyes 86

Face 93
Face X-rays 48
Facial nerve innervation 94f
Failed airway and back-ups 73
False negatives 17
False positives 17
Family 110
Family history 2
FDIC 128
Felon 98

Entrapped foreskin 82

Femoral 78, 94
FENa 30
Fetal monitor 83
Fever 5, 93
Fiberoptic 72
Finance and savings 128
Fines 110
Finger and nail bed cut-away 98f
Fingers 90, 92
Fingertip 96
Flare of chronic Dz 102
Flex-Ex 48
Fluoresceine 86
Fontanelle 5
Foot 52
Foot peripheral nerves 13
Foreign bodies 51, 87, 93
Foreign language emergencies 3
Foreign language translation resources 3
Foreskin procedures 82
Formulae 5, 30
Fracture reduction anesthesia 92
Fractures 48, 92, 102
Framing 101
Fraud 120
Free air 50
Free fluid behind bladder 54f

G-tubes 81
Gall bladder wall 57
Gallstone and pericholecystic fluid 57f
Gallstone in neck of gallbladder 57f
Gallstones 57
Gasping 131
Genitourinary 82
Getting along with others 123
GFR 30, 31
GI scans 65
Glabelar 14
Glasgow Coma Scale 14t
Glucagon 136
Glucose 31, 41, 85, 137
Goals for nurses 124
Good Samaritan law 117
Gram stain 85
Greenstick 51

Hand 51
Hand-offs and transitions in care 109
Hand peripheral nerves 12
Hand washing 6
Hand zones 96f
Hands and feet 96
Hawthorne effect 121
Head CT 62
Health 126
Health insurance portability and
   accountability act 110
Heart 55f
Hematoma 87
Hematoma block 92
Heme 41
Hemoglobin 36
Hemoglobin A1c 33
Hemoglobin changes 36
Hemolytic 36
Hemorrhage 83
Hemostatis 39f, 95
Hemothorax 54
Herpes 44
High-risk symptoms and standards of care 102t

Highlights of critical care drugs 136
Himalayan T-waves 28f
Hip 52, 89, 91
History of ED ultrasound 53
History taking in a foreign language 3
HMOs and denial of care 120
Holding orders 106
Home and after-care instructions 103
Homeless patients and EMTALA 108
Horner's causes 10
Horner's syndrome 8
Hydrocephalus 62
Hydronephrosis 57f
Hygroma 62
Hyperkalemia 24
   junctional rhythm 28f
   peaked T-wave 28f
Hypertrophic obstructive
   cardiomyopathy 25
Hypomagnesemia: Large U-wave 28f
Hypomagnesemia: QT prolongation 28f
Hypotension 135
Hypothermia 5, 24
Hypothermia with Osborne J-waves and
   shiver artifact 24
Hypoxemia 4t

"I PREPARED" for documentation of
   procedure 69
Idioventricular rhythm 24
Imaging in pregnancy and ACOG
   recommendations 47
Immunologic tests 43
Impaired driving and DMV notification 105
IMR 120
In-procedure considerations 99
Inamrinone 136
Incision and drainage 98
Incomplete history 101
Incorporation 128
Incorporation bias 121
Induced hypothermia and post-arrest
   care 133
Induction agents 71t
Infections 25, 36, 93, 102
Informed consent 69
Informed refusal 69
Informed refusals for admitted
   patients 107
Infusion Rx 120
Ingrown toenails 98
Injecting anesthesia 93
Internal jugular 78
Intra-oral 93
Intraosseous lines 79
Intubation 72, 131
Intussusception 58
Invasive 17
Investment 128
Involuntary admissions 107
Irrigation 86
Ischemia 21–22, 25, 64
Ischemic changes classification on
   EKG by location 21t
Ischemic EKG by the Sgarbossa criteria 22f
IV contrast 61
IVC 55

J-point 19
Jaw 90
Job search and interviewing 125

Joint Commission 127
The Joint Commission and site surveys 127
Jones fracture 52f
Junctional rhythm 24f
Junctional tachycardia 26

Ketones 31, 32
Kidney 57
Knee 52, 89, 91
KOH 44
KUB/abdominal series 50

Lab 30–44
Lab adjustments 17
Lab formulae 20
Labeling 101
Lacerations 93–97
Lactate 31, 32
Lateral canthotomy 86
Laying on of hands 6
LBO 50
LDH 34
Left kidney with spleen and diaphragm 57f
Leg peripheral nerves 13
LET/XAP 93
Leukemia 37
Leukocyte esterase 41
Levine sign 8f
LFTs/GI 30
Lidocaine 79, 136
Lifelong learning self assessment 127
Light wand 73
Likelihood ratio 122
Lines 137, 139
Lip/mouth 97
Lipase 34
Literature review 121
Lithium 40
Litigation threat 116
Liver function tests 34
LMA 73
LMX-4 93
Long QT interval 25
Lost revenue 120
Lower extremity 52
Lumbar puncture 84
Lumbar spine 50
Lumbar spine CT 63
Lung and chest wall injuries 75
Lung sounds 11t
LV assist device 131

Macrocytic 36
Magnesium 31, 136
   high, low 28
Making a diagnosis 101
Malaria 43
Malpractice insurance 117
Mandatory reporting 111
Mandible 48
Mandible relocation 90f
Meckel's 65
Meconium 139
Med-legal 117–118
Medical board investigations 125
Medical decision making 120
Medical literature 121–122
Medication 132
Meta-analysis 122
Metabolic acidosis 32t
Metabolic alkalosis 32t

Metamyelocytes 37
Metastases 50, 62
Metformin 61
Methylene blue 89
Metoprolol 136
MI and LBBB 22
MI and pacer 22
MI and RBBB 22
MI/ACS 102
Microcytic 36
Milestones 1
Mini-Mental Status Exam 14t
Minors 110
Miosis 10
Mixed acid-base disorder decoding 33
Mobitz I 24, 132
Mobitz II 24, 132
Mold 92
Monocytes 38
Morrison's pouch/RUQ 54f
Motor 14
Moving air 131
MRI 47, 63
MRI in ED 67
MRI of spinal epidural abscess
    missed by CT 67f
Mucous retention cyst 62
Multifocal atrial tachycardia 26
Murmurs 11t
Muscle compartments 88t
Mydriasis 10
Myocardial infarction onset 35f
Myoglobin 35

Nail bed 96
Nasal foreign body 87
Nasotracheal 72
National practitioner data bank 117
National Stark Law 120
Neck—soft tissue X-rays 48
Negative predictive value 122
Neonatal critical care drug dosing 138t
Neonatal resuscitation 139
Neonate 85
Nephropathy 61
Nerve 96
Nerve blocks 94
Neuro exam 14, 16f
NEXUS tool 48
NG tubes 81
NIH stroke scale 15t
Nitrites 41
Nitroprusside 136
Nodules 49
Noncompressible DVT 60f
Non-pressor agents 135t
Nor-Epi 136
Normocytic 36
Notice of intention to sue 117
NTG 136
Nuclear medicine tests 65
Number needed to harm 122
Number needed to treat 122
Nurses 124
Nurses interactions 114
Nystagmus 10, 14t

Obese 18
Observational bias 121
Observational studies 121
Obstetrics/gynecology 59, 83

Occam's Razor 129
Ockham's oversight 101
Odds ratio 122
Odontoid 48
Office f/u 108
OLD CARTS 1
Open joint 89
Opiates 105
Organ donation 109
Organ donor 134
Ortho 51, 120
Ortho exam 12, 13
Ortho pitfalls and misses 51
Osmolality 30
Osmolality gap 30, 40
Osteomyelitis 51
Ovaries 59
Overconfidence 101

P wave 19
Pacing 132
Packing 87
Padding 92
Pain ease 93
Paint guns 96
Palliative care 109
Palmonetal 14
Pancreas plus 34
Paperclips 86f
Paracentesis 81
Paraglossal 72
Paralytic agents 71t
Paraphimosis 82
Parasitic infection 25
Parsimony 101
Past medical history 2
Past surgical history 2
Patella 91
Patella relocation 91f
Pathogenic, urine culture 41
Patient and family interactions 113
Patient satisfaction 129
Patients in police custody 111
PE 102
PEA 132
Peaked T-wave 20
Pediatric airways 73
Pediatric critical care drug dosing 138t
Pediatric exam 5
Pediatric history 1
Pediatric resuscitation 137
Pediatric vascular access 77
Pediatric vital signs 5t
Pediatrics 51
Peds 18
Pelvic CT 64
Pelvis 52
Peptide Nucleic Acid Fluorescence in
    Situ Hybridization 43
Pericardial tamponade 76f
Pericardial tamponade with
    RV collapse 55f
Pericardiocentesis 77
Pericarditis 18f
Peripheral IV tricks 77
PGE1 136, 137–138
pH 17
Phalen's test 8f
Phosphorus 31
Photography 110
Physical exam 4–16

Physical exam summary chart 6
Physician order for life-sustaining
    treatment form 109
Physician Quality Reporting Initiative 106
Physician wellness 126
Placenta 83
Plaster 92
Platelet function test 38
Platelets, high, low 38
PMDs interactions 114
Pneumatosis intestinalis 50, 64
Pneumothorax 11, 18, 54
Pneumothorax aspiration 75
Poking technique 79
Police 110
Polymerase chain reaction 43
Poor man's exercise stress test 23
Population studies 121
Portal air 64
Post-anesthesia and pre-repair 95
Post-arrest care 134
Post-hoc analysis 122
Post intubation checklist 74
Post-procedure 69
Post-procedure considerations 99
Post-repair care 97
Posterior epistaxis 87
Positive predictive value 122
Potassium 18, 31
Potassium, high, low 28
PPD 43
PR interval 25
Precipitants 1
Pregnant 18
Premature closure 101
Premature ventricular contractions 27
Presedation considerations 99t
Present on admission 120
Press-Ganey scores 126
Press-Ganey scores and
    expectation management 113
Pressor 135
Pressors comparison 135t
Pre-test likelihood of
    coronary disease 23t
Pretreatment agents 70t
Prevention and documentation 116
Priapism 82
Prinzmetal 21
Prior visit 1
Pro time 34
Procedural sedation 99
Procedures 69
Professionalism and keeping your job 125
Prolactin 34
Pronestyl 136
Protein 41, 85
Pseudo MI 21
Pseudosac 59
Psych meds 29
Psychiatric holds 107
PT 38t
PTT 38t
PTT goals for heparin therapy 38t
Publication bias 121
Pulmonary anatomy 11f
Pulmonary edema and hypotension 135
Pulmonary embolism 18
Pulmonary nodule 49
Pulmonary V/Q scans 65t
Pulse ox 4, 120

Pulse pressure 4
Pulseless arrest 137
Pulseless V-tach and V-fib 132
Punctures 96
Pupillary findings 10f
Pupils 10

Q-wave 19
QRS axis 19
QRS voltage 19
QRS wide 19
QT long 20
QT short 20
Quantiferon 43
Queckenstedt's test 84
Quitting 126

Radiation 17, 45–46
  doses 47
  risks 45
  risks from diagnostic imaging 45–46
Rapid ultrasound in shock and
  hypotension protocol 55
RBCs 41, 85
Recall bias 121
Records 46
Red flags 101
Red herring 101
Reducing substances 41
Reflexes 5, 14
Refusals 104
Regional anesthesia, to extremities,
  face 94
Relative benefit 122
Relative risk 122
Renal function tests 31
Renal stone 64
Repair
  of face and head 97
  general 95
  of hands and feet 96
Reperfusion 21
Respiratory rate 4
Restraints 107
Results reporting 122
Resuscitation 131
Retics 36
Retrograde UrethroGram 82
Retropharangeal abscess 63f
Reversal agents 71t
Review of systems 2
Rhythm 18
Ring removal 96
Risk for various diseases per unit of blood
  transfused 36t
Risk management 113–116
Risks of tests 17
Ristocetin cofactor 38t
RSR' 18
RSTUVW 7
Rules for being pimped 129
Rules for the emergency medicine
  resident 129
Rules for the internal medicine
  resident 129
Rules for the surgical resident 129
Ruptured ectopic with clotted blood 59f
RV dysplasia 25

S1S2S3 18
S-wave 19

Salter Harris 51f
SBAR 123, 127
SBO 50
"SCAB CHANT" 74
Scabies 44
Scalp 97
Schedules 128
Screening 2
Search satisfied 101
Sedation 120
Seeing Red 129
Seidel's test 86
Selection bias 121
Sensitive 110
Sensory 4
Sensory nerves of dorsal and
  palmar hand 12f
Sensory nerves of lower leg 13f
Septal hematoma 87
Septic 137
Serology 43
Sestamibi 23
Severe hyperkalemia with
  sine waves 24f
Severity by Salter Harris 51f
Sexual assault 111
Sexual harassment 125
Sgarbossa positive 22
Shock 55, 137
Shock and pressors 135
Shock types and management 135t
Short PR 25
Shoulder 51, 89, 90
Sick Sinus Syndrome 26
Significance 122
Sinus bradycardia 24
Sinuses 62
SIPC 128
Site choice 78
Skin microscopy 44
Skull X-rays 48
Small bowel obstruction 64
Small parts and procedures 59
Smoking gun 101
SOAP MIRA 70
Social history 2
Sodium 31, 41
Soft tissue neck CT 63
Soft tissues 50
Some basic insurance needs 14
Specimens collection 30t
Spectrum 46t, 101
Spectrum bias 121
Spin 122
Spinal cord 16
Spine 14, 50, 63
Splinting 92, 97
Splints 92
Sponsorship bias 121
SQ fluids 7
ST depression from toxic
  digoxin level 29f
ST-normal 19
Staff interactions 114
Staples 95
STD testing 44
Steeple sign 48
Steri-strips 95
Sterno-clavicular joint 90
Steroid injections for bursitis and
  tendonitis 88

Stigmata 25
Stool culture 42
Stool guaiac card 42
Stool: Infection 42
Stop test 23
Straw man 122
Stress echo 23
Stress tests 23
Stroke 62, 102
Study considerations 121
Study design types 121
Study interpretation 122
Study methods 121
Subclavian 78
Subdural empyema 62f
Subpoenas 117
Subungal hematoma
  trephination 98
Supra-ventricular tachycardia 26
Suprapubic view 54f
Surrogate markers 122
Suture talk 96
Suture type comparison 95t
Suturing 95
Swan-Ganz 78
Syncope 111
Syncope or palpitations 25
Syphilis 44

T3 and T4 34
T-V1 wave 22
T-wave 20
TAC 93
Tachycardia 4, 25, 137
  narrow 26
  narrow with a pulse 133
  wide 27
  wide with a pulse 133
Tachydysrhythmias 133t
Tagged RBC scan 65
Tagged WBC scan 65
Tarasoff 111
Teamwork in ED 123–124
"Ten Commandments" of
  Emergency Medicine 101
Tendons 96
Test characteristics 122
Test results 114
Testicular 65
Tests 17
Tetanus/dT 93
Theophylline 40
Thoracentesis 75
Thoracic spine 50
Thoracic spine CT 63
Thoracotomy 75
Throat 87
Throat culture 42
TICLES 5
Tiers of nursing care
  sophistication 124
Time out and universal protocol 69
Toe/finger 89
Tongue 87
Topical anesthetics 93
Torsade 27
Torsion 59
Tourniquet 77
Tox 30
Toxic granulation 37f

Toxicology testing 40
Transfers 108
Transfers in 108
Transfers out and the homeless 108
Transfusions 36
Transthecal 94
Trauma 54, 62, 64, 131, 137
Traumatic rupture of
    the aorta 63
Trephination 98
Triads of diseases 8t
Triage bias 101
Trial and cross examination 118
Troponin 63
Troponin I 35
TSH 34, 62
Tubes 137, 139
Two-point discrimination 12
Tylenol level 40t
Tzanck 44

U-wave 20
Ultrasound 53–60, 79, 94
    jugular vein anatomy 79f
    for peripheral IVs 77
Uncertainty 101
Units 46
Upper extremity 51
Urethrograms 82

Urine culture 41
Urine dip 41
Urine micro 41
Urine tox 40
Urology 59

V fib 132
V leads 18
V/Q scans 94
Vaginal bleed 59
Vaginal delivery 83
Valecula sign 48
Valproate 40
Varices 81
Vascular and DVT 60
Vascular labs 35
Vascular ultrasound 66
Vasopressin 136
Veins of arm 77f
Venous cutdown 80
Venous gas 32
Ventilation 131, 134
Ventilator management 74
Ventilators 32
Ventricular tachycardia 27f, 132
Vessels 48
VF/VT 137
Viral infection 25, 42
Vital sign decoding 4–5

Vocal cords 71f
VP shunt tap 84

Wall motion 55
Waves and intervals 19–20
Wax 87
Ways to fool the reader 121
WBC, high, low 37
WBCs 37, 41, 85
Weeks/See 59
Wellen's warning 22
Wide SVT 27
Wire 78
WNL 38, 83
Wolff-Parkinson-White 25f
Woods lamp 44
Workers' comp dictation 103
Workers' compensation discharges 103
Workup bias 121
Wound culture 42
WPW 27
Wrist 51, 89, 90
Wrist band 127

X-rays 47–52, 120
Xanthochromia 85

Z-puncture 81
Zavanelli 83